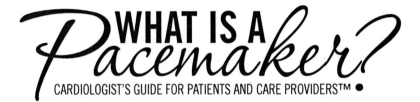

WHAT IS A *Pacemaker?*

CARDIOLOGIST'S GUIDE FOR PATIENTS AND CARE PROVIDERS™ ●

Dr. JEFFREY L WILLIAMS

ISBN: 1481916602
ISBN-13: 9781481916608
Library of Congress Control Number: 2013900670
CreateSpace Independent Publishing Platform
North Charleston, South Carolina

Disclosure: The information and images included in this book are for educational purposes only. It is not intended nor implied to be professional medical advice or a substitute for professional medical advice. The reader should always consult his or her healthcare provider to determine the appropriateness of the information for their own situation or if they have any questions regarding a medical condition or treatment plan. Reading the information in this book does not create a physician-patient relationship. Trademarks, product names, or logos featured or referred to in this book are the property of the trademark or logo holders and are used for informational purposes only. Images and patient scenarios have been altered for purposes of anonymity and are used for educational purposes only.

Acknowledgements: To my wife and three great kids without whose never-failing patience (and sometimes frustration) I would have never completed this book. To my patients who tolerate my furious pace and bad jokes.

Table of Contents:

CHAPTER 1
Introduction:

The hectic pace of today's doctors has shortchanged the information-sharing process for patients undergoing pacemaker implantation. Patients and their families are often unaware of many critical issues involved in pacemaker implantation. Though pacemaker implantation can usually be performed with minimal risks, any surgery entails risks that are particular for each procedure and patient. I have found it increasingly difficult to provide a complete consultation, physical exam, and discussion about the risks, benefits, and alternatives of pacemaker implantation in a typical forty-five-minute session. Since starting the Heart Rhythm Center in 2008, I have developed several iterations of written and online patient-education materials to complement our office discussions. This book serves as a comprehensive summary of the steps involved with pacemaker implantation: from the initial evaluation and implant procedure to the possible postoperative complications and required long-term follow-up care for patients and their caregivers (both professional and laypeople alike). Furthermore, many of my extremely elderly patients rely upon their spouses and families for help with the decision-making process and long-term care of their device. This book serves as a thorough means to ensure that all family members understand the roles, risks, and required follow-up for pacemaker patients.

Approximately 140,000 patients currently undergo pacemaker implantation in the United States each year.[1] As the burgeoning population of baby-boomers age, this is expected to grow to almost two hundred thousand pacemakers per year by 2030.[2] In addition, the elderly are the most rapidly growing segment of the United States,[3,4] and pacemakers are commonly implanted in this population. There are reports of pacemaker implant complications—generally clinical trials reporting outcomes and incident complication rates—and fewer reports of complication rates in the extreme elderly (with a persistent exclusion of elderly patients from ongoing clinical trials).[5]

This is the first and only book dedicated solely to patients, families, and their care providers as a comprehensive review of the "what, why, and how" of pacemaker implantation. As our patients become more and more invested in decisions that affect their health care, more detailed information is necessary so patients can make a comprehensive assessment prior to proceeding with any surgical procedure. This book can be part of the informed-consent process, because it covers more thoroughly the entire pacemaker implantation process than can be presented in a single (or even multiple) office visit(s). A particular emphasis will be placed on the complications that can occur during/after pacemaker implantation and how to assess a particular pacemaker implanter's odds of a successful operation. Finally, patients concerned that they may need a pacemaker will find this book a useful summary of the complete evaluation that is performed to see if a pacemaker may be of benefit.

CHAPTER 2
Basics of Heart Anatomy and Conduction System:

Blood flow through the heart. Figure 1 depicts the basic structure of the heart. Blood returns from the body and enters the right atrium. The blood leaves the right atrium through the tricuspid valve, and it enters the right ventricle. The right ventricle then pumps the blood through the pulmonary valve into the lungs. The blood is oxygenated in the lungs and is returned to the left atrium. The blood leaves the left atrium through the mitral valve and enters the left ventricle. The left ventricle pumps the oxygenated blood through the aortic valve to the rest of the body; it then returns to the heart via the right atrium.

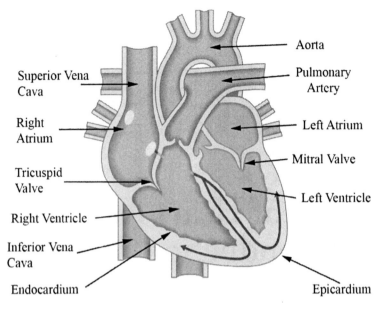

Figure 1: Basic Anatomy of the Heart

If the coronary arteries of the heart represent the "plumbing," then the conduction system of the heart represents the "wiring." **Figure 2** represents the conduction system of the heart. Normal heart rate is sixty to one hundred beats per minute (bpm). Bradycardia is an abnormally slow heart rate less than 60 bpm, and tachycardia refers to an abnormally fast heart rate greater than 100 bpm. The sinoatrial (SA) node serves as the internal clock—or native pacemaker—of the heart and signals the appropriate heart rate for a given situation.

Electrical conduction system of the heart: The heart's natural pacemaker (the SA node) is located in the top right chamber of the heart: the right atrium. The SA node sends a signal to the upper chambers (the right and left atria) and the lower chambers (the right and left ventricles) via the atrioventricular (AV) node. The AV node transmits the electrical signal to the bottom chambers via the left and right bundle branches. The left bundle branch is comprised of left posterior and left anterior fascicles. "Fascicles" is another term for divisions or branches. Often, the patient has a slow heart rate because the electrical connection between the top (the signal from the SA node) and bottom (the ventricles) of the heart is diseased, called AV block. The most common type of pacemaker involves placing leads in the right atrium and right ventricle.

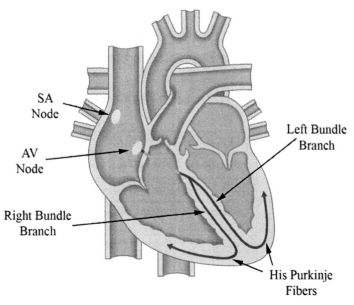

Figure 2: Conduction System of the Heart

Coronary arteries: The coronary arteries supply blood (and hence, oxygen) to the heart muscle and course along the outside of the heart (epicardium). Each coronary artery supplies particular muscle territories in your heart. The left main coronary artery comes off the aorta and branches into the left anterior descending (LAD) and circumflex (CX) arteries. The right coronary artery (RCA) comes off the right side of the aorta and ultimately branches into the posterolateral (PLA) and posterior descending arteries (PDA). See **table 1** for blood supplies of various elements of the conduction system. One can see why AV Block is often seen during heart attacks (blocked coronary artery) involving the RCA, because 80% of patients have their AV node blood supply provided by the RCA. In addition, left posterior fascicular block is uncommonly due to coronary disease, because it has a dual blood supply. It would require two occluded coronary arteries (PDA and LAD septal perforators) to become blocked.

Table 1. Blood Supply to the Heart's Electrical Conduction System

STRUCTURE	BLOOD SUPPLY (% OF PATIENTS)
SA Node	55% RCA; 35% Left Circumflex; 10% Dual
AV Node	80% RCA; 10% Left Circumflex; 10% Dual
RBB	LAD Septal Perforators, AV Nodal Branch of RCA
LBB: LAF	LAD Septal Perforators
LBB: LPF	PDA and LAD Septal Perforators

-SA=sinoatrial, AV=atrioventricular, RBB=right bundle branch, LBB=left bundle branch, LAF=left anterior fascicle, LPF=left posterior fascicle.

Electrocardiogram: One of the most important tools that doctors have to assess the electrical function of your heart is the electrocardiogram. **Figure 3** depicts a typical electrocardiogram tracing and shows how this waveform represents the electrical and pumping actions of your heart. The P wave corresponds to the electrical activation of the right and left atria. The right and left atria contract and pump the blood to the right and left ventricles, respectively. The PR interval is the time it takes for the electrical activation from the SA node, through the AV node, to the right and left ventricles. The QRS complex is the electrical representation of the right and left ventricle contracting and pumping blood out of the heart. The T wave corresponds to repolarization (or resetting of the ventricles' electrical system) prior to the next contraction of the heart.

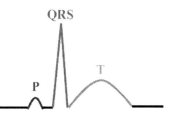

1. Atrial Contraction (P)
2. Ventricular Contraction (QRS)

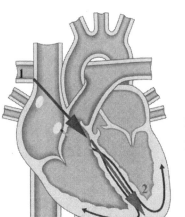

Figure 3: The Electrocardiogram and Its Relation to Heart Timing/Pumping

CHAPTER 3
Reasons for Pacemaker Implantation:

Introduction. Your care providers have extensive training assessing the reasons—also called indications—that a patient may need a pacemaker. In particular, it is very important that the benefits of pacemaker implantation outweigh the risks of the pacemaker implant surgery (to be discussed later). The American College of Cardiology (ACC) is one of the major professional societies that develops guidelines to help care providers make educated clinical decisions that are based upon prior clinical studies. This is the basis of "evidence-based" medicine: the process by which clinical ideas are tested, reported, and reevaluated to decide the most appropriate care for a particular condition.

The ACC has developed guidelines that help care providers decide when a patient would be best served by a pacemaker.[6] The easiest rule to remember is: *pacemakers are most appropriate for patients who are having symptoms related to an abnormally slow—or at times, fast—heart rate.* These symptoms include: shortness of breath, chest pain, dizziness, fainting (also called syncope), heart failure, arrhythmias (such as ventricular tachycardia/fibrillation), or fatigue.

The decision to implant a pacemaker also requires evaluation of the permanence of the AV block. Electrolyte abnormalities (like potassium) can cause significant AV block, but correction of the abnormality can lead to resolution of the AV block. Some diseases—like Lyme Disease—often follow a natural course where the AV block is temporary and resolves as the disease is treated. Some types of AV block that occur during periods of vagal activation can reverse very quickly (e.g., nausea and dizziness during a blood draw may cause transient AV block or during sleep in patients with sleep apnea). In addition, after aortic valve surgery, inflammation can cause transient AV block that resolves within days of the operation. Finally, there are some diseases that warrant pacemaker implantation, because the AV block may continue to worsen (for example, sarcoidosis, amyloidosis, or neuromuscular diseases).[6]

Pacemakers for slow heart rates (bradycardia) due to sinoatrial and atrioventricular node dysfunction.

Sinoatrial node dysfunction. The sinus node is the heart's pacemaker—or metronome. As patients age, the pacemaker may beat too fast, and this can be treated with medicines that slow the heart rate. These medicines include beta blockers, such as: metoprolol, atenolol, propranolol, or carvedilol. More often, however, sinus node dysfunction can cause the heart to beat too slowly. A patient can be symptomatic, because the heart is beating too slowly (symptomatic bradycardia) or does not beat fast enough during exercise (chronotropic incompetence). In situations where the heart does not beat fast enough or where medications to treat fast heart rates cause the heart to beat too slowly, a pacemaker can be used to reestablish a normal heart rate.

> _Common clinical scenario:_ An eighty-year-old woman on no medications has progressive symptoms over the last one to two years, including: fatigue, shortness of breath, and an inability to walk far with a heart rate not exceeding 100 bpm. She has an echocardiogram (sonogram of the heart) and nuclear stress test that are normal. In the office, she is walked on flat ground and one flight of steps, and she is short of breath with a maximum heart rate of 80 bpm. She is exhibiting symptoms and clinical findings that suggest chronotropic incompetence from sinoatrial node dysfunction.

In my practice, I find a surprising number of patients who have been experiencing symptomatic chronotropic incompetence. As a person exercises, he or she is more and more dependent upon heart rate to increase the amount of blood that is pumped by the heart (cardiac output). A rule of thumb is that a person's maximum heart rate is 220 minus their age. There are several ways to assess chronotropic incompetence: (1) inability to achieve maximum heart rate, (2) delay to reach maximum heart rate, (3) inadequate submaximal heart rate or recovery heart rate, and (4) excessive variation in heart rate during exercise (rate instability).[7] Chronotropic incompetence has been found in 11–26% of patients undergoing stress tests, and it is associated with an increased risk of death—likely associated with underlying coronary artery disease.[8]

Acquired atrioventricular block in adults. The most important thing to remember is: a pacemaker is most beneficial when a patient has symptoms attributable to conduction delay through the AV node. AV block refers to conduction delay between the top (atria) and bottom (ventricles) chambers of the heart. There are several different types of AV block, and these include: first-degree AV block, second-degree AV block, and complete heart block. First-degree heart block represents a simple delay in the AV node; it is generally harmless and does not require a pacemaker. Second-degree heart block occurs when electrical impulses are intermittently blocked between the atria and ventricles. It can be a normal, nonfatal finding in patients (e.g., Type I second-degree AV block) but can also cause symptoms and may require a pacemaker (e.g., Type II second-degree AV block). Third-degree AV block (also called complete heart block) occurs when the electrical connection between the atria and ventricles is disrupted, and the chambers beat independently with no electrical connection. *Most often, third-degree heart block requires a pacemaker.*

> *Common clinical scenario: A sixty-year-old male has an abrupt loss of consciousness while at church and is brought to the emergency room. The EKG shown below is obtained. His electrolytes are normal. The EKG shown below depicts the atrium (P waves) beating at 80 bpm and the ventricles (QRS complexes) electrically disconnected from the atrium and beating independently at 35 bpm. This is an example of third-degree, or complete, heart block. He underwent a successful pacemaker implantation.*

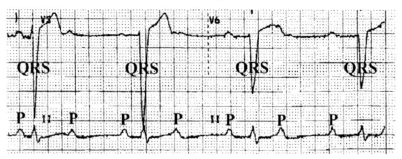

Chronic bifascicular block. Bifascicular block refers to block below the AV node in the right and left bundle branches. The left bundle branch is comprised of the left posterior and left anterior fascicles. A person can have alternating right and left bundle branch and this patient is at risk of complete heart block; pacemaker implantation is generally recommended. Patients with bifascicular block and evidence of complete heart block or second degree AV block will likely benefit from pacemaker support. Patients that present with syncope (fainting) and bifascicular block often undergo an electrophysiology (EP) study to evaluate the conduction system. The results of this EP study may suggest that the patient is at risk of complete heart block and he or she may benefit from a pacemaker.

> _Common clinical scenario:_ A seventy-two-year-old male with a history of coronary artery disease and coronary artery bypass grafting comes to the ER with multiple episodes of fainting. His workup suggests that the only abnormality is bifascicular block, based on his ECG. He undergoes an EP study, where several catheters are placed in his groin and guided up the leg veins into his heart. Evidence of conduction system disease below his AV node is found. This type of disease is called His purkinje system disease, and in the setting of bifascicular block, places him at risk of abrupt episodes of heart block that can cause him to faint. He undergoes a pacemaker implantation.

Atrioventricular block associated with acute myocardial infarction. Patients who have heart attacks (called acute myocardial infarctions) may require pacing support. Most often, this pacing support is temporary and is removed within one to two days of the heart attack. Sometimes, a patient has preexisting ECG abnormalities and continues to have issues with symptomatic slow heart rates or heart block after the heart attack; this patient may require a permanent pacemaker.

Hypersensitive carotid sinus syndrome. Hypersensitive carotid sinus syndrome is also known as carotid sinus hypersensitivity (CSH). CSH is an extreme reflex response to carotid sinus stimulation: rubbing the carotid artery where it runs next to the Adam's apple. There are two components of the reflex:[6] (1) cardioinhibitory response, resulting from increased parasympathetic nervous system tone, is manifested by a slowing of the sinus rate or prolongation of the PR interval and advanced AV block—alone or in combination, and (2) vasodepressor response, which stems from a reduction in sympathetic nervous system activity that results in loss of vascular tone and hypotension (drop in blood pressure) independent of heart rate.

It is very important to determine if a patient has the cardioinhibitory response to carotid sinus stimulation when deciding if a pacemaker implantation is warranted. A pause of more than three seconds—causing low blood pressure or fainting—is suggestive of CSH. Pacemaker implantation in patients with excessive cardioinhibitory response to carotid sinus massage is usually effective at relieving symptoms. CSH in elderly patients is also associated with carotid vascular disease,[9] and it may be associated with 45–50% of elderly patients that present with falls.[10,11]

> *Common clinical scenario: An eighty-two-year-old female with a history of falls is admitted to the hospital after a recurrent unexplained fall—causing a hip fracture. Her workup is normal, but a carotid sinus massage results in an approximately-eight-second pause pause on hospital telemetry (as shown below). She undergoes pacemaker implantation and experiences no further falls.*

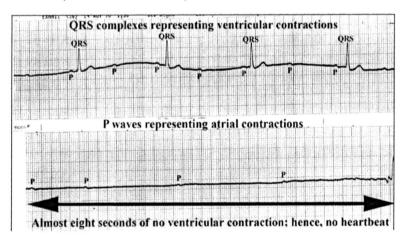

Neurocardiogenic syncope: Neurocardiogenic syncope (also called vasovagal syncope) comprises a variety of clinical presentations resulting from a neural reflex that causes peripheral arteries to relax and lead to low blood pressure (hypotension). This reflex may also cause an abnormally slow heart rate (bradycardia). It presents with a prodrome (set of symptoms occurring together)

that often consists of: dizziness, nausea, vomiting, or diaphoresis (sweating). It is important to note that these prodromes may be absent in the elderly. They are often situational, and they can occur with: pain, stress, bowel movements, blood draws, or prolonged standing. There is generally no evidence of heart disease, and pacing is rarely indicated. Recurrent episodes of syncope (especially without warning symptoms)—refractory to noninvasive management strategies such as medicine, compression hose, or situational avoidance—may be treated with permanent pacing. Sometimes, a patient may undergo a Tilt Table Test to evaluate causes for syncope. This involves placing a patient on a table that tilts up to a steep angle and watching for blood pressure and heart rate changes that cause symptoms.

Miscellaneous reasons for pacemaker implantation. The most common reasons for pacemaker implantation were discussed in the preceding paragraphs, but there are other situations in which pacemakers may be necessary.[6]

Patients who have had heart transplants may have slow heart rates (bradycardia) that respond to pacing.

Neuromuscular diseases—such as muscular and myotonic dystrophies—may cause progressive conduction system disease, leading to complete heart block. Even asymptomatic patients may benefit from pacemakers—depending upon other risk factors such as abnormal electrocardiograms or electrophysiology studies.

Patients with sleep apnea (breathing stops during sleep) may have slow heart rates (sinus bradycardia) or even long pauses while sleeping. Rarely is pacemaker therapy required for these heart rhythm disturbances.

Sarcoidosis causes granulomas (abnormal collections of immune cells) to form that have heart involvement in 25% of patients, and heart block may develop in 30% of these patients. Depending upon the clinical situation, patients with sarcoid may benefit from pacemaker support.

Pacemakers can be used for the prevention and termination of heart rhythm abnormalities. A variety of atrial and ventricular arrhythmias can be prevented and terminated by a pacemaker. In particular, patients with long QT syndrome may benefit from pacemakers, because many rhythm disturbances are initiated by slow heart rates; more often, however, these patients require defibrillators to prevent sudden death.

Atrial fibrillation is a common rhythm disturbance that requires pacemaker support. The vast majority of atrial fibrillation patients require medicines to slow down their heart during periods of atrial fibrillation. There are patients who have atrial fibrillation with very slow heart rates, or the medications used to control the fast heart rates (tachycardia) during atrial fibrillation lead to very slow heart rates (bradycardia) when normal rhythm returns. This is called tachycardia-bradycardia syndrome. These patients with atrial fibrillation may benefit from pacemaker placement.

There are situations where a pacemaker is placed because of "hemodynamic" reasons. "Hemodynamics" refers to the pumping of blood through the heart and vascular system. Sometimes, patients with heart failure will benefit from a special pacemaker that resynchronizes the heart (to be discussed later). Also, patients who have abnormal heart muscle thickening (hypertrophic cardiomyopathy) may require pacing to help treat their condition.

Finally, a pacemaker may be required in children, adolescents, and adults with congenital heart disease (or heart defects they were born with).

Summary. The most common indications for permanent pacemaker implantation have been discussed, including typical case scenarios. Obviously, not all patients "read the textbooks," and their symptoms may be atypical and may have findings that overlap several categories; therefore, it is critical to have an open dialogue with your care providers. There are other conditions that may warrant pacemaker implantation such as: cardiac transplants, systemic disease (like sarcoidosis and neuromuscular disorders), and even sleep apnea. I always recommend that patients get a second opinion if they are uncomfortable with a treatment plan or have rare disorders.

CHAPTER 4
What are Pacemakers, and How Do They Work?

Location of pacemaker implantation. The most common implant location is underneath the left collar bone (called the clavicle). There are two reasons for this: (1) the majority of patients are right-handed, and placing the device on the left minimizes risk of damaging the patient's dominant arm; and (2) a pacemaker implantation is technically less demanding when placed on the left side. Pacemaker leads are placed into veins that drain the arm and lead back to your heart. The two major veins in your arm are the cephalic (shown in **figure 4**) and the basilica vein. These join to form the axillary vein, which then forms the subclavian vein (shown in **figure 4**). This venous structure is found in both arms—though sometimes people have anatomic variants.

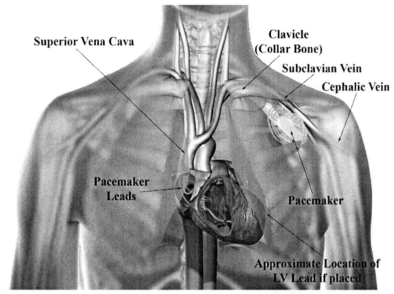

Superior Vena Cava

Clavicle
(Collar Bone)

Subclavian Vein

Cephalic Vein

Pacemaker
Leads

Pacemaker

Approximate Location of
LV Lead if placed

Figure 4: Configuration of Pacemaker and Lead Implants. (Reproduced with permission of Medtronic, Inc.)

The incision is about five to eight centimeters (one to three inches) long, and the device pocket is made under the skin but above the chest muscle. The leads are placed into the subclavian vein and ultimately, into the heart. Once the leads are placed into the heart, they are then sewn into place and connected to the pacemaker. The pacemaker is placed into the device pocket—with the remaining portion of the leads coiled under the pacemaker—and the pocket is then sewn shut. Generally, the pacemaker (see **figure 4**) is placed just under the left (shown) or right collar bone.

Common clinical question: Is there a difference between pacemakers and defibrillators? All defibrillators are pacemakers, but pacemakers are NOT defibrillators. Defibrillators also involve placing leads into the right atrium and ventricle. These leads can also be used to prevent the heart from beating too slowly (i.e., they can function as a pacemaker), but they have an additional role. The defibrillator lead in the right ventricle allows the device to sense a possibly fatal arrhythmia. If a fatal arrhythmia is detected by the device, it can shock the patient back to life! This is very similar to what you see on TV, except there are no paddles applied to the chest wall; the device leads permit us to deliver over seven hundred volts directly to the inside of a patient's heart. Again, all defibrillators are pacemakers, but pacemakers are NOT defibrillators.

What are the elements of a pacemaker? The pacemaker itself is comprised of a battery, circuitry that serves as the brain, and the header that is used to connect the leads to the pacemaker itself. **Figures 5A, 5B, and 5C** show: typical sizes of pacemakers (**5A**), basic lead types (**5B**), and internal construction of a pacemaker (**5C**).

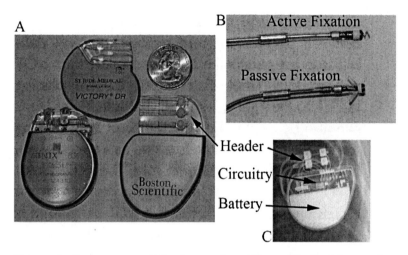

Figures 5: Components of the Pacemaker (Sizes of Typical Pacemakers (A), Lead Types (B), and Pacemaker Construction (C)) The different sizes of pacemakers are shown compared to the size of a quarter. (5A) Active and passive fixation leads are shown. (5B) An X-ray showing the cross section of a pacemaker with battery, circuitry, and header to attach leads. (5C)

The majority of the size of the pacemaker is due to the size of the battery and header. The headers can vary in size depending upon the number of leads attached to the pacemaker; a pacemaker with a single lead has a smaller footprint than a pacemaker with three leads attached. The two types of leads are called active and passive fixation. Fixation describes how the pacemaker lead is attached to the heart. **Figure 5B** shows an active fixation (screw) and passive fixation lead (silicone tines). The active fixation lead is comprised of a tiny screw that is rotated to engage the inner wall of the heart (endocardium). This is the most common type of lead implanted in the right atrium and ventricle. The passive fixation lead has soft plastic "barbs" called "tines" at the tip; these tines anchor the tip of the lead to the heart. There are many intricate "nooks and crannies" that line the inside of your heart (called trabeculations). These trabeculations allow passive fixation leads to anchor in place. These leads are not as common, because they can be technically challenging to implant. There is some evidence that these passive fixation leads are safer in extremely elderly patients, because they are less likely to cause a perforation (hole in the heart). All current left-ventricular leads used in the heart-failure pacemakers (resynchronization devices) are passive—except for one model (Starfix™, Medtronic Inc., Minneapolis, MN) that has a mechanism to prevent dislodgement.

Pacemaker to help heart-failure patients. Patients receiving pacemakers may be at risk for, or even have, heart failure. They can have dyssynchronous contraction (the right and left ventricles do not pump at the same time) that causes heart failure symptoms such as: shortness of breath and leg swelling. This may require an additional lead to be placed into the coronary sinus that can pace the left side of your heart (the left ventricle). This lead in the left ventricle is used to "resynchronize" the pumping action of the heart so that the right and left ventricles pump at the same time. The coronary sinus is paper thin, very easily perforated, and requires great care and caution to implant. Indeed, left ventricular leads can be technically demanding to implant, and they may add hours to a pacemaker implant. **Figure 4** also shows the approximate position of a lead (LV lead) that is used to pace the lower left chamber of the heart (called the left ventricle).

How are pacemakers programmed? Your care providers communicate with your pacemaker to give and get information via a wand placed over the device or wirelessly (now available on most devices). A programmer is used to check the device to make sure the leads are functioning properly and to program pacing features on the pacemaker. This is called interrogation. Pacemakers are "programmed" to pace, depending on the condition the doctors are trying to treat. **Table 2** describes the different modes that your pacemaker may be programmed to. Pacemakers can be programmed to pace at different rates determined by your doctor. There is also a way to program your pacemaker to pace at a rate that matches your activity level. This is called "rate-responsive" programming.

Table 2. Different Programming Modes of Pacemakers

MODE OF PACING	LEADS REQUIRED	HOW DOES IT WORK?	CLINICAL SCENARIO
Single-chamber (Atrial)	Right-atrial lead	This will only pace your atrium if the rate falls below the programmed cutoff (usually 40–60 bpm).	A 60-year-old male with sinus node dysfunction and chronotropic incompetence with no other conduction system disease
Single-Chamber (Ventricular)	Right-ventricle lead	This will only pace your ventricle if the rate falls below the programmed cutoff (usually 40–60 bpm).	80-year-old female with permanent atrial fibrillation who passes out from slow heart rates (bradycardia)
Dual-chamber	Right-atrial and -ventricular lead.	This can pace your atrium and/or ventricle if the rates fall below the programmed cutoff (usually 40–60 bpm).	56-year-old male who fainted and was found to have complete heart block because of underlying coronary artery disease
Biventricular	Right- and left-ventricle +/- right-atrial lead.	This can pace your atrium (if needed) and ventricles. Because the goal of this device is to resynchronize your heart, both the right and left ventricles are always pacing.	70-year-old male who has very symptomatic heart failure and an abnormal electrocardiogram

CHAPTER 5
Preoperative Workup and Evaluation (Meeting the Implanting Physician):

Introduction. The first important element of the evaluation for a pacemaker is the type of doctor who will be performing the pacemaker implantation. All doctors have years of training built upon a foundation of patient evaluation that permits a thorough, yet concise, summary of a patient and his or her symptoms, medical history, and differential diagnosis. The differential diagnosis consists of the possible diagnoses (in order of likelihood) that can explain the patient's symptom constellation. That being said, there is a wide variety of doctors (and training backgrounds) who can implant pacemakers.

- A *cardiologist* is an Internal Medicine doctor whose training involves four years of undergraduate college, four years of medical school, three years of Internal Medicine residency, and three years of Cardiology fellowship. Many cardiologists are board-certified in Internal Medicine and Cardiology.

- An *electrophysiologist* (EP) is a subspecialized cardiologist who performs heart-rhythm evaluations and electrophysiology device implants, such as: pacemakers and defibrillators. Typical training involves the same training as a cardiologist— plus an additional two years of Electrophysiology (Heart Rhythm) fellowship. During this Electrophysiology Fellowship, an EP focuses exclusively on pacemaker and defibrillator implantation as well as long-term care of these devices. In addition, an EP is trained in all aspects of heart-rhythm evaluation and care: including electrophysiology studies and heart ablations to cure various arrhythmias. Many EP's are board-certified in Internal Medicine, Cardiology, and Clinical Cardiac Electrophysiology.

- *General and cardiothoracic surgeons* can often implant pacemakers; and some can implant defibrillators. Surgeons undergo five years of a general surgery residency and heart surgeons will do an additional two to three years of heart surgery.

Their training involves the implant procedure with no long-term follow-up pacemaker care (except in few instances). Oftentimes, pacemakers need to be implanted during open-heart surgery. In other cases, general surgeons at community hospitals implant pacemakers, because the cardiologists are not trained to perform implantation.

I have seen cardiologists, electrophysiologists, and surgeons with exceptional (and catastrophic) outcomes of pacemaker implant surgery. There are *several questions you can ask the implanting physician* to assess his or her chances of a successful pacemaker with low risk of complications.

QUESTIONS TO ASK YOUR DOCTOR BEFORE SURGERY

1. What is your training background?

There is evidence that physician training (specifically, board-certification or board-eligibility in clinical cardiac electrophysiology) may result in lower rates of complications such as lead dislodgement.[12,13]

2. How many have you done?

Doctors who perform more pacemaker implants seem to have fewer complications than doctors who only perform a handful a year. Specifically, higher-volume (greater than twelve implants per year) versus lower-volume operators (fewer than twelve implants per year) have also demonstrated lower rates of complication.[14]

3. What have your complications been?

This question can be especially enlightening, because it will give you an idea if this doctor has looked at his or her outcomes. A doctor who tells you he or she has no complications is misinformed or has not done enough procedures. Any doctor that performs procedures has complications, and a doctor that cares about patient outcomes will have done due diligence to minimize complications from happening again. That being said, there is generally no way to have zero complications, but it is important to choose a doctor that has in-depth knowledge of possible complications.

4. What type of pacemaker will be implanted, and why?

A rule of thumb is that more complex devices (dual-chamber vs. single-ventricular-chamber pacemakers) have been associated with higher rates of complications. However, there is also data that does not demonstrate increased rates of complications in dual-chamber devices.[16] In addition, the placement of a left-ventricular lead may entail more time and risk than other types of leads.

History of present illness (HPI). The most important element of evaluating a patient is an open discussion to determine the "present illness." It is estimated that over 80% of patients can be diagnosed just by obtaining an accurate history from the patient.[15] One of the most important aspects in the evaluation of a patient for a pacemaker is whether or not the patient has symptoms that are associated with abnormally fast or slow heart rates. Symptoms such as loss of consciousness (or syncope), dizziness, shortness of breath, chest pain, palpitations, or exertional fatigue can all be related to heart rhythm disorders requiring a pacemaker.

Typical Patient HPI: This is a seventy-two-year-old white female that has had eleven episodes of sudden loss of consciousness over the past four years. She has had witnessed seizure activity, and under the care of her primary care physician, neurologist, and general cardiologist, she has been started on an anti-seizure medicine. She continues to experience these episodes of syncope. Each episode involves a short period of dizziness and eyes blacking out. This is followed by a loss of consciousness. These episodes, more often than not, are abrupt in their onset, occur without much warning, and have resulted in injury at times. They can occur while seated or standing. They do not appear related to meals, dehydration, emotional stress, or any other obvious cause. There are no related symptoms such as chest pain, shortness of breath, or rapid heart beat.

Common elements of the history of present illness (HPI): We can boil the HPI into seven categories to encompass all elements of the history. "COLDER-AS" is a mnemonic used to ensure that I ask all the right questions when evaluating a patient: Character, Onset, Location, Duration, Exacerbating Factors, Relieving Factors, and Associated Symptoms (see **table 3**).

Character concerns the subjective elements of the symptom or problem. Each of the remaining elements is then used to describe the particular issue for a complete description. The HPI can be gathered from anyone familiar with patient care. Physician extenders—such as nurse practitioners, physician assistants, nurses, or medical assistants—may gather this background information. It is not so much how the information is obtained; rather, that *all* the information is obtained.

Table 3. Major Elements in the History of Present Illness

<u>C</u>haracter	Pressure, burn, ache
<u>O</u>nset	Circumstances/timing of symptoms
<u>L</u>ocation	Where is the pain felt, and is it felt in any other locations?
<u>D</u>uration	How long have the symptoms been present and how long do they last?
<u>E</u>xacerbating factors	What has the patient done to aggravate the symptom (walking, sitting, standing, eating, drinking, etc.)?
<u>R</u>elieving factors	What has the patient done to relieve the symptom (deep breathing, cold water, nitroglycerin, belching, aspirin, etc.)?
<u>A</u>ssociated <u>S</u>ymptoms	What are the symptoms that the patient notices to occur at same time as the main issue? (Examples include: shortness of breath, heart racing, sweating, nausea, vomiting, etc.)

Past medical and surgical history (PMH). The past medical and surgical history helps to "risk stratify" patients. Elements of a patient history—including prior heart attacks (myocardial infarction or MI), congestive heart failure (CHF), or arrhythmias such as ventricular tachycardia/fibrillation and atrial fibrillation—suggest underlying heart disease and possibly higher rates of conduction-system disease. In fact, there are other noncardiac medical problems that can hint at a possible cardiac condition that may indicate the need for a pacemaker. Peripheral vascular disease (blockages in arteries such as your carotids in the neck or arteries in the legs) can also indicate that heart disease is present. Not only can coronary arteries get plaques (or fatty blockages), the heart's conduction system can also be diseased by the buildup of calcification or fibrous scar tissue.

Social history. The "social" history is used to obtain details of a person's life that are not purely medical. Personal habits such as the use of tobacco (causing vascular disease), alcohol, and illicit drugs—which are toxic to the heart muscle and cause heart rhythm abnormalities—raise the suspicion of serious heart problems. Additionally, personal stresses—such as deaths in the family, marital issues, or the loss of a job—can increase stress. Many heart-rhythm abnormalities are exacerbated by: increased stress, decreased sleep, caffeine, alcohol, or nicotine. Conversely, regular exercise, a healthy diet and sleep habits, smoking cessation, and weight loss can decrease heart rhythm abnormalities.

Allergies. Obviously, your doctors should be aware of any drug allergy or prior concerning reaction to any medication. Often the first exposure to a medication causes a minor reaction, but the second exposure can lead to a fatal allergic reaction (called anaphylaxis). It is also important to let your doctor know if you have any reactions to other substances. Knowing of a prior reaction to intravenous contrast agents (such as during a CT scan or cardiac catheterization) or latex gloves can enable your doctors to avoid using these agents or give prophylaxis so an adverse reaction is minimized. Prophylaxis may include the use of steroids and antihistamines. Steroids such as prednisone or hydrocortisone are often used preoperatively. In addition, antihistamines like diphenhydramine (also called Benadryl™) and famotidine (also called Pepcid™) are given to reduce the severity of a possible allergic reaction.

Family history. The saying: "an apple does not fall far from the tree" is used to emphasize the importance of family history. We are trained to specifically ask for family histories of heart disease—and the age at which they occurred. The relative must be a blood relative (not an in-law), and we are mainly concerned with first-degree relatives: such as mother/father or sister/brother. That being said, even aunts, uncles, and cousins may have medical problems that can be inherited by the patient. Common heart problems that can be transmitted from generation to generation include: coronary artery disease, heart attacks, atrial fibrillation, and sudden deaths.

Sudden death refers to an unexpected (and sometimes at a very young age) death that was likely related to the heart.

Additional family histories that may suggest sudden cardiac deaths include "unexplained" seizure disorders or drownings in relatives who knew how to swim. During a sudden cardiac death, the heart muscle stops pumping, causing the brain to experience a lack of oxygen and possible seizure. Family members that have sudden cardiac deaths (and miraculously recover in seconds) may be misdiagnosed with seizure disorders. In addition, some conditions that can cause sudden cardiac death are triggered by vigorous exertion (e.g., long QT syndrome); if this person was swimming when a sudden cardiac death occurred, the death may be mistakenly called a drowning.

Physical exam (including vital signs). Vital signs include: heart rate (heartbeats per minute), blood pressure, respiratory rate (breaths per minute), and pulse ox (pulse oximetry measures the oxygen content of blood).

Heart rate: A normal range of resting heart rates is sixty to one hundred beats per minute (bpm). Bradycardia refers to a heart rate less than 60 bpm, though sometimes, very physically fit people can have normally slow resting heart rates less than 60 bpm. Tachycardia refers to a heart rate more than 100 bpm. Generally, your heart rate accelerates to 100–120 bpm during a brisk walk or steps (called sinus tachycardia), and this is a normal response to exercise. An abnormally slow response to exercise—the inability to get heart rate above 100 bpm with associated chest pain or shortness of breath—can indicate sinus node dysfunction and is called chronotropic incompetence. Abnormally fast heart rates can indicate abnormal heart rhythms that need medical treatment. The following box describes a very common arrhythmia that can result in significant heart-rate variation.

What is atrial fibrillation?

Atrial fibrillation (AF) is the most common arrhythmia seen in a typical electrophysiology practice and often presents with an abnormal or irregular heart rate. Almost 5% (5 out of 100) patients aged greater than sixty years have AF, and it increases almost 0.5% per year until by eighty years of age, up to 15% of people may have atrial fibrillation.

AF refers to the top chambers of the heart (the right and left atriums) fibrillating (or beating rapidly) at 300–400 bpm. This rapid beating is transmitted to the lower pumping chambers of the heart (ventricles) and causes most of the symptoms attributed to AF, such as: palpitations, heart racing, chest pain, or shortness of breath. The most concerning aspect of AF—aside from the aforementioned symptoms—is the risk of stroke (blood clots sent to the brain). AF causes the atrium to stop contracting and just quiver. This loss of pumping can lead to blood-clot formation in the atrium. The diagnosis of atrial fibrillation (or atrial flutter, a closely related heart rhythm disorder) should lead to a discussion with your doctor about anticoagulation to prevent the development of strokes.

Blood pressure: The goal blood pressure in most patients is 120/80. The top number is called the systolic blood pressure, and the bottom number is called the diastolic blood pressure. When a patient has elevated blood pressure, diet and exercise can often normalize blood pressure. Sometimes, diet and exercise are not enough, and most doctors treat blood pressures above 140/90 with medication. Recent research suggests that extremely elderly patients (age greater than eighty years) may have a higher target blood pressure.

Respiratory rate: The respiratory rate refers to how often a person breathes in one minute. The normal rate is approximately eight to fourteen breaths per minute. Shortness of breath (or difficulty breathing) is often associated with an increased respiratory rate.

Pulse oximetry: Pulse oximetry is used to determine the oxygen saturation in the blood. Normal oxygen saturation is greater than 95%. Sometimes, heart patients can have abnormal (low) pulse oximetry readings due to the presence of heart failure (or COPD).

Weight: Weight is important to obtain, because patients who have heart failure will often gain weight. Close monitoring of weight can allow a patient to alert his or her doctor of an impending heart-failure exacerbation. Generally, rapid weight gain (or loss) of more than two to three pounds in several days corresponds to fluid weight. In addition, abnormally high or low body weights may place a patient at a higher risk of pacemaker implant complications.

What is Congestive Heart Failure?

Congestive heart failure (CHF) generally means that your heart cannot pump blood as efficiently as your body needs it to. This is most commonly due to the heart's weakening and its inability to pump enough blood (called systolic heart failure). CHF often occurs when a patient's ejection fraction (EF) drops below the normal of 55–70%. In addition, a common type of heart failure (called diastolic heart failure) results from an inability of the heart to relax properly. Diastolic heart failure is common in elderly patients with high blood pressure. Symptoms of heart failure include:

- Shortness of breath during exertion or while lying down
- Chest pain
- Swelling (edema) in feet, ankles, or legs
- Irregular or fast heart rate
- Weakness and fatigue
- Reduced ability to walk or exercise
- Coughing (sometimes with pink sputum) or wheezing
- Sudden weight gain
- Loss of appetite or stomach discomfort

—New appearance of these symptoms should be relayed to your doctor.

Pertinent studies. There are many tests that the implanting physician will want to obtain prior to pacemaker implantation. A *chest radiograph* (also called, chest X-ray) is obtained to ensure that the lungs and heart are in suitable condition for pacemaker implantation. In addition, the baseline chest X-ray will be used as a comparison to determine if there has been any complication from the pacemaker implantation. The *electrocardiogram* (EKG) is obviously obtained to evaluate for any heart-rhythm disorders or electrical-system blockages. An echocardiogram (echo for short) is used to assess for any decline in heart-pumping function (ejection fraction) as well as to assess for heart chamber sizes and any valve disease. *Stress tests* may be performed prior to proceeding with pacemaker implantation. Reasons for stress tests include: (1) to see if symptoms such as chest pain or shortness of breath are due to underlying coronary artery blockages, or (2) to assess an adequate heart-rate response to exercise. Finally, *baseline blood laboratories*—such as kidney function, blood counts, and blood coagulation studies—are performed to make sure the pacemaker implantation can be performed safely.

Preoperative risk assessment. As with all surgical procedures, recognizing and managing existing medical problems (aka, comorbid conditions) preoperatively helps to mitigate the risks during and immediately after pacemaker implantation. The association of heart failure and other structural heart disease with cardiac conduction-system disease—as well as the expanding role of biventricular pacemakers specifically indicated for patients with symptomatic congestive heart failure—means that there is an inherently high risk population of patients frequently served in the EP lab. Indeed, CHF increases the risk of all surgery. A decreased ejection fraction (EF) has been found to be a predictor of peri-operative complications, with the highest risk group being those with an EF less than 35%: the very patients brought to the lab for resynchronization pacemakers. Pre-procedural management of CHF is integral to the safety of the procedure. Patients certainly should not be in a state of decompensated heart failure.

Infection.[16] Patients who present with systemic infection and positive blood cultures carry the highest risk of infection.[17] Infection of implantable devices is one of the most feared complications due to the dismal prognosis of untreated infections and risk of device removal. Often, we are asked to evaluate patients for bradycardias (slow heart rates) when they happen to be identified at the time of hospitalization for infectious etiologies—such as pneumonia and urinary tract infections—as well as post cardiac surgery. Pre-implant evaluation for potential sources of infection is critical. The estimated rate of infection of permanent pacemaker leads is between 1 and 2%; however, the range is from under 1% to greater than 10%. Device infection requiring removal was correlated to fever within twenty-four hours of device implant, temporary pacing prior to implant, and early reintervention for lead revision or hematoma evacuation.[18] The likelihood of infection was nearly doubled by the patient having undergone placement of a temporary pacemaker. The association with temporary intravenous pacing wires certainly implies an association with any indwelling lines—including central lines and PICC lines. The duration of hospitalization prior to implant was not correlated to higher risk of infection. Infections were generally not related to new pacemaker implantation and perioperative antibiotic prophylaxis. Believe it or not, the use of perioperative antibiotics is considered controversial; although, I routinely use post-operative antibiotics for five days after pacemaker implantation.

Use of contrast agents during pacemaker implantation.[16] Bones show up very well on X-rays; however, soft structures (such as blood vessels and the heart) are not well visualized on X-ray. Contrast refers to a clear liquid that is used to highlight blood vessels and heart structure during pacemaker implantation. The implanting physician will use fluoroscopy to guide the implant procedure. Fluoroscopy is a special type of imaging that allows us to perform X-rays while the patient or the heart is moving. Fluoroscopy allows us to watch catheters and leads moving in the blood vessels and the heart so that we can place them in the correct location. A typical use of contrast for a pacemaker implantation is during a subclavian venography. Subclavian venography is done to ensure that a person's subclavian vein is not blocked so that a pacemaker can be implanted safely. If we encounter a blocked left subclavian vein on venography, we can change the implant to the right side prior to making an incision.

Contrast-induced nephropathy (CIN). Contrast-induced nephropathy (kidney failure) is a surprisingly common complication if radiocontrast is given during a procedure; CIN can occur in 15% of cases. It is a decline in kidney function (by checking the blood level of creatinine) and typically peaks at forty-eight to seventy-two hours after exposure. Creatinine may remain above baseline for seven to fourteen days. Naturally, the best way to avoid this complication is to abstain from its use. Single- and dual-lead pacing systems can safely be implanted without the use of contrast at all. Prior data from our Heart Rhythm Center[19] revealed that contrast was used in fifty-five of ninety-two (59.8%) of the pacemaker implantations with a mean intravenous contrast usage of 9.6cc. No contrast was used for generator changes, and there were no contrast reactions. Cardiac resynchronization therapy (CRT) device implantation for heart failure may require contrast agents to define the coronary sinus (CS) anatomy. CS lead placement can be performed successfully without the use of contrast in patients at risk of contrast-induced nephropathy.[19]

The vast majority of patients undergoing CRT implants are patients with heart failure and its associated comorbidities—which very frequently include diabetes and chronic kidney disease. Therefore, a working knowledge and respect for these agents is a necessity. There are several things I do to limit the danger of kidney damage: (1) use a very weak, diluted contrast agent, (2) aggressively hydrate the patient (especially those with kidney disease at baseline); hydration can usually be achieved with four to six glasses of water the evening before the procedure, and (3) hold medications that can worsen kidney damage during the procedure (for example, ACE inhibitors, angiotensin receptor blockers, and NSAIDS can be held the day prior and day of exposure and be resumed twenty-four hours after exposure), and medications such as sodium bicarbonate and N-acetylcysteine (Mucomyst®) are given prior to pacemaker implantation. Treatment of CIN is largely supportive (generally resolves on its own) and infrequently requires short-term dialysis.

Contrast allergies. Immediate life-threatening allergic (anaphylactic) reactions—including angioedema (facial and throat swelling), bronchospasm (lung spasm), arterial hypotension (low blood pressure), and shock—can occur within minutes of and up to sixty minutes after injection of IV contrast.[20] The reported incidence of severe immediate reactions to ionic contrast material (CM) is 0.1–0.4%, and with the newer, non-ionic, and low osmolar or iso-osmolar contrast, it is 0.02–0.04%. But death rates from the two materials do not differ.[21] Patients with even mild anaphylactoid (immediate) reactions should be considered high risk in future contrast administration.

It is common practice to pre-medicate with corticosteroids with or without histamine (H1) blockers (e.g., Pepcid®) in patients with a history of moderate or severe immediate reactions—despite the fact that randomized trials comparing pretreatment strategies are severely lacking. Prior to any procedure that may involve contrast administration, *it is essential that you inform your doctor about any history of previous contrast reaction, asthma, renal insufficiency, diabetes, and metformin therapy.*[22] Routine pre-medication of all patients who receive contrast is probably not warranted given the overall low incidence of a reaction; in fact, some have advocated abandoning this procedure altogether.[23] Patients with a history of severe contrast allergy who will likely need IV contrast during a procedure should probably receive pre-exposure treatment with corticosteroids (such as prednisone or hydrocortisone) as well as H1 blockers—although strong evidence of benefit is lacking.[24] If contrast administration cannot be delayed for four to six hours after steroids, some would omit use and administer only H1 blockers.[22] Weaker agents—such as low-osmolar or iso-osmolar contrast such as ioxaglate, iohexol, or ioversol—should be used due to the lower overall incidence of reactions in patients with a history of asthma or a contrast allergy. The specific contrast agent causing the prior reaction should be sought and avoided if possible, although this information is often difficult for your doctor to obtain. Despite pretreatment with steroids and H1-blockers, reactions are still possible in those with prior reactions.

Thyroid Issues.[16] Hypothyroidism (low thyroid function) has been found in 0.5–0.8% of the population: demonstrated by elevated serum levels of thyroid-stimulating hormone (TSH) or decreased serum thyroxine levels.[25] Undiagnosed (hence, untreated) hypothyroidism can lead to major perioperative complications including: severe hypotension (low blood pressure) or cardiac arrest following induction of anesthesia, extreme sensitivity to narcotics and anesthetics with prolonged unconsciousness, and hypothyroid coma following anesthesia and surgery.[25] Ideally, hypothyroidism is caught early and thyroid supplement (thyroxine) administered until the patient's thyroid function has normalized—generally, four to six weeks.

Hyperthyroidism (high thyroid function) affects approximately 0.2% of men and 2% of women and may cause atrial fibrillation, congestive heart failure, and thrombocytopenia (low blood cells).[26] In addition, anesthetic drugs may be affected by the hypermetabolic state of hyperthyroidism. When total intravenous anesthesia is used—often at our center this occurs when high frequency jet ventilation is used to minimize respiratory motion—an increased dose of sedatives may be needed, because these agents are processed more quickly with a hyperactive thyroid.[26,34]

Generally, more thyroid-related perioperative complications stem from hypothyroidism as opposed to hyperthyroidism; however, recognition of either prior to implantation is important. Our Heart Rhythm Center

CHAPTER 6
The Implant Procedure:

Registration and check-in. Patients generally undergo pacemaker implantations at the hospital and require an overnight stay. Rarely do patients go home the same day as an implant, although this can happen. Some doctors operate at multiple hospitals, so it is important to make sure at which hospital the procedure is to be done. The patients will generally check in with registration and then go to the appropriate *holding area* (preoperative or "preop" unit). This is a staging area where the patient changes into a gown, an IV is started, and hospital documentation is performed. At this time, the patient is asked multiple times his or her name and the type of procedure that is to be performed. Questions often seem redundant—e.g., Do you have any allergies? What surgery are you here for?—but this fact-checking is an attempt to minimize any chance of medical error. Most implanting doctors will meet their patient here to answer any last-minute questions and confirm that all preoperative tests are complete and the surgery can proceed.

Informed-consent process. The informed-consent process is one of the most important aspects of any medical procedure. It is more than just getting a patient to sign the consent form. This is the process by which a patient is informed of the diagnosis and the nature and purpose of the proposed treatment or procedure. The patient should understand the risks and benefits of the proposed pacemaker implantation as well as the risks and benefits of any alternative treatments, such as medications or watchful waiting. Obviously, this book can be part of the informed-consent process, because it covers more thoroughly the entire pacemaker implantation process than can be presented in a single (or even multiple) office visit(s). It is during this process that patients can ask questions to be sure they fully understand the rationale for the pacemaker and can ask questions they might have for the physician. Some physicians go over these risks, benefits, and alternatives in the office and have the patient more thoroughly review and read the consent form at home prior to the pacemaker implantation. Once the patient has completed the required elements in the holding area and the informed consent process is completed, he or she is brought into the *procedure room*.

The procedure room. The procedure room may be a standard operating room or may be a specialized cardiac-catheterization laboratory (where heart catheterizations are usually performed) that has been altered to perform pacemaker implantations. It is here that one of the most important parts of the procedure is performed. A *time out* is when the doctors, nurses, technologists, and all personnel that are participating in the surgery stop what they are doing (before the patient is sedated) and identify the patient, the procedure being performed (including site of implant), the technique to be used, and any other important patient information (such as drug allergies). Again, the time out is performed to minimize the occurrence of any medical errors—like placing a pacemaker in the wrong patient!

At this point in time, the procedure can be started. Most patients are sedated for the pacemaker implantation. Conscious sedation involves giving medications that relax the patient and relieve pain but allow the patient to breathe on his or her own. Conscious sedation can be administered by nurses in the room or by anesthesiologists. General anesthesia involves deep sedation: often requiring a temporary breathing tube and connecting the patient to an artificial ventilator. General anesthesia is administered by anesthesiologists or specially trained nurses: called certified registered nurse anesthetists (CRNAs). The choice of anesthesia is usually at the discretion of the implanting physician. Oftentimes, the higher the risk of the surgery, the more often general anesthesia is used. In my opinion, general anesthesia permits for tighter control of patient heart rate and blood pressure and allows the patient to remain absolutely still during the procedure. These elements may permit a safer procedure as well as a more pleasant experience for the patient.

The implant procedure. The implant procedure is performed under sterile conditions in an operating room or cardiac procedure room that includes sterile supplies, a patient table that is adjustable, and an X-ray system called fluoroscopy. **Figure 6** shows a typical implant procedure room. The C-arm holds the X-ray equipment that the physician uses to guide pacemaker wires into the correct positions; this technique of using X-rays to guide implantation is called fluoroscopy. The screens display patient information—like EKG and blood pressure—and show the X-ray images. The anesthesia equipment and anesthesiologist are at the head of the bed. A special sterile table holds all the instruments and equipment that will be used during the implantation.

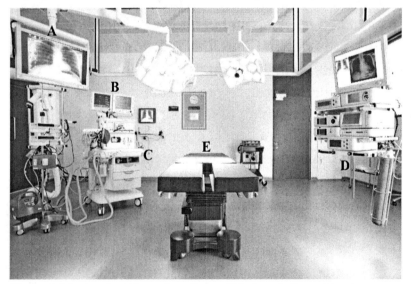

Figure 6: The Implant Procedure Room This is a dedicated implant procedure room that includes: X-ray equipment to permit lead placement (A), screens displaying patient information (B), anesthesia equipment (C), equipment to program the newly implanted pacemaker (D), and the patient table (E).

The components of a pacemaker are described in **chapter four**. Most pacemakers are placed under the left collarbone. Most patients are right-handed, so left-sided implants are preferred. There are two reasons for this: (1) it is technically less-demanding to place pacemaker leads from this location, and (2) Any complications that occur are worse if they occur on the side of the patient's dominant arm. The most common access site is the left subclavian vein (or axillary vein). Oftentimes, more experienced implanters can perform a left cephalic vein cut down. This approach has been associated with fewer complications: such as pneumothorax, hemothorax, or lead fractures. I generally attempt left cephalic cut down on patients at high risk of complications: such as extremely elderly patients (age greater than eighty years) or very small patients (weighing less than one hundred pounds).

The incision location is generally located two finger breadths below the clavicle. It is important to note that the ultimate location of the incision and device may vary considerably—depending upon patient size. I may place an incision two finger breadths below the clavicle during the surgery, but when the patient wakes and stands up, he or she may see considerable shift of the chest wall tissue that causes the device to be substantially lower. This shifting of the incision and pacemaker can be seen in both obese and thin patients.

Operative Steps of Pacemaker Implantation

1. Sterile preparation and draping of the patient occurs on the operating table.

2. Patient is sedated.

3. Specialized personnel prepare the implant area under the right or left collarbone and cover the rest of the patient with sterile gowns.

4. Implanting physician sterilely scrubs hands for several minutes then puts on sterile gown and gloves.

5. Lidocaine is used to numb the skin, and a one- to three-inch incision is made.

6. Device pocket is made under the skin but above the chest wall muscle. This pocket will hold the pacemaker and any extra lead material.

7. The subclavian vein is punctured with a needle, and a wire is placed through this needle. The needle is withdrawn—leaving the wire in the vein. Over this wire, a hollow tube is placed, and the pacemaker lead is placed through this hollow tube. Once the lead is attached to the heart, the hollow tube is removed, and the lead is sewn in place to the chest wall muscle. This is repeated for each pacemaker lead.

8. The leads are tested to be sure they are functioning well and then attached to the pacemaker.

9. The pacemaker is then placed into the pocket with the leads coiled underneath. The incision is then closed with several layers of sutures. The top layer of skin may be closed with staples or Steri-Strips™.

10. Sterile dressing is placed, and the patient is wakened from sedation and returned to the recovery area.

Immediately post-implant. Once the patient is awake with no obvious complications, he or she is generally observed in the hospital overnight. In our Heart Rhythm Center, patients are kept lying in bed for four hours after the implantation. They can eat once they are awake and alert after the procedure. We keep a sterile dressing on the wound until the next morning when we examine the incision. Some centers perform a chest X-ray immediately after the implantation. However, if the patient has had no obvious implant complications, I obtain a chest X-ray (CXR) the next morning to verify that the leads are still in the correct position. A typical post-implant CXR is shown in **figure 7**. We use this post-implant chest X-ray to verify correct lead position and assess for complications. I have included an overlay of the heart's anatomy to give you an idea of heart chamber locations.

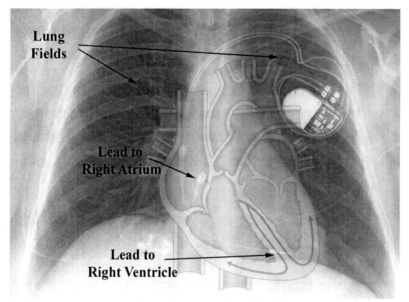

Lung
Fields

Lead to
Right Atrium

Lead to
Right Ventricle

Figure 7. The Basics of Reading a Chest X-ray. This is a typical post-implant chest X-ray—with superimposed cartoon of the heart to show you *approximate* location of cardiac chambers—used to verify correct lead position and assess for complications. Your cardiologist uses the CXR to make sure that the leads are in the correct chamber of the heart. We normally look for damage to the lungs and lead positions after the implant is completed.

Day after the implantation. The morning after the implantation, the sterile dressing is removed and the incision is inspected by the doctor, nurse or an assistant. I leave a layer of butterfly stiches (Steri-Strips™) over the incision; generally, the incision can be left without a gauze dressing—as long as the incision care instructions in next section are followed. If there is any oozing, a clean, dry gauze can be placed over the incision to protect clothing from blood staining. Finally, the device is "interrogated," using a special bedside computer called a programmer. **Figure 8** shows a mock interrogation being performed. Usually an electronic wand is placed over the pacemaker site, and this is used to exchange information with the pacemaker. The programmer is used to check the lead functions and send any programming changes to the pacemaker. Generally, patients do not feel any symptoms during device checks and programming, though occasionally, a patient can notice different heart rates during the check. Once the pacemaker is interrogated, any changes are saved onto the pacemaker, and the patient is ready to go home.

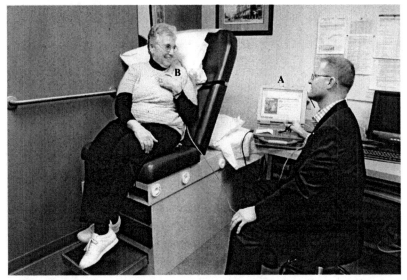

Figure 8: Device Interrogation. This shows a typical office visit for a pacemaker check (called interrogation). The programmer (A) has all the software necessary to check and program the pacemaker. Many pacemakers allow wireless interrogations but many still require a wand (B) that is held over the pacemaker to communicate with the device

CHAPTER 7
Possible Complications of Device Implantation:

Introduction. This section is written for both patients and primary care doctors, though it is a bit more complex than the rest of the book. In most cases, I have attempted to boil the complication rates down to simple percentages and show the imaging that I use to detect these complications. It will familiarize patients with the names of common complications and how we detect and treat them. I strived to provide the best image of a particular complication—In some cases, the device pictured is a defibrillator rather than a pacemaker. In addition, it is heavily referenced to demonstrate the basis for the estimated rate of complications and provide physicians with further reading material. For a more detailed discussion on complications of pacemaker implantation that Dr. Robert Stevenson and I co-authored, please see: http://www.intechopen.com/books/current-issues-and-recent-advances-in-pacemaker-therapy/complications_of_pacemaker_implantation.[16]

Figure 9 shows the incidence of complications that can occur during pacemaker implantation. Major and minor complications can occur in approximately 4–7% of patients within thirty days of pacemaker implantation.[16,27,28] This means that for every one hundred patients that undergo a pacemaker implantation, four to seven patients may experience a major or minor complication. The diamond shows the average rate that the complication occurs as a percentage; the bars depict the range of complication rates that is possible. For instance, leads become dislodged an average of 2.3% of the time as reported in prior trials, although it can vary from 0.5–4% of the time—depending upon the implanting physician.

Major complications have been defined as: death, cardiac arrest, cardiac perforation, cardiac valve injury, coronary venous dissection, hemothorax, pneumothorax, transient ischemic attack, stroke, myocardial infarction, pericardial tamponade, and arterial-venous fistula. Minor complications have been defined as: drug reaction, conduction block, hematoma or lead dislodgement requiring reoperation, peripheral embolus, phlebitis, peripheral nerve injury, and device-related infection. One of the major techniques we use to evaluate for complications from pacemaker implantation is the chest X-ray (also called chest radiograph). **Figure 7** shows a typical chest X-ray of a patient after undergoing a pacemaker implantation. The pacemaker device is placed in the left upper chest and leads are seen in the right atrium and right ventricle. One can see the lung fields, cardiac silhouette, ribs, and diaphragm. The chest X-ray can be quickly assessed for lead position and damage to the heart or lungs.

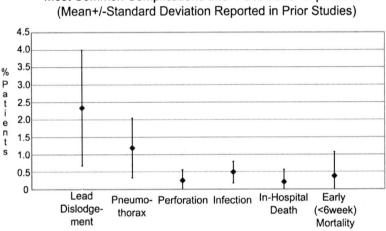

Figure 9: Most Common Complications after Pacemaker Implantation (Figure originally published by Williams and Stevenson[16])

Complications that can occur prior to going home.

Sedation/Airway: Less than 20% of electrophysiology (EP) programs in the United States exclusively use anesthesia professionals for procedural sedation.[29] Minor complications (e.g., atelectasis or minor lung compression, fever, or vascular congestion) may simply be reflective of common postoperative pulmonary complications (PPC) seen after general anesthesia. Atelectasis can be seen on CT scan in up to 90% of patients who are anesthetized[30] and PPCs have been found to occur in 9.6% of patients.[31] There is data to suggest that patients undergoing invasive EP procedures may require deep conscious sedation that often is converted to general anesthesia;[32] thus, the use of general anesthesia (including high frequency jet ventilation to minimize patient movement) during EP procedures may enhance patient safety.[33,34]

Pneumothorax: Pneumothorax may occur in as many as 3–4%[35,36] and as few as 0–1%[16,19] but generally ranges from 1–3% of patients undergoing pacemaker implantation.[14,27,28] A pneumothorax is a collection of air outside the lung but underneath the lung lining (pleural space). It can cause the lung to collapse. It is caused by damaging the lung during lead placement and is often more common in smokers or extremely thin patients. Routine chest radiographs may be performed immediately after pacemaker implantation, though clinical signs of pneumothorax include: low oxygen on pulse oximetry, shortness of breath, pleuritic pain (pain that is worse with deep breathing), and low blood pressure. **Figure 10** depicts the radiographic appearance of small, medium, and large pneumothoraces. Emergent treatment of pneumothorax includes decompression of the pressure built up by the air collection. This decompression is done by placing a tube through the chest wall to drain the air collection (called pleurocentesis). This can be done by the implanting physician, but it is usually performed by a surgeon. Oftentimes, high concentrations of inspired oxygen can lead to a resolution of a small pneumothorax (comprising less than 30% lung volume).[37] This conservative treatment of pneumothorax can reduce further complications and duration of hospitalization and avoid invasive drainage procedures. The traditional treatment of patients with traumatic (e.g., motor vehicle accidents) hemo- or pneumo-thoraces has been an insertion of a chest tube (CT). CT have larger caliber than smaller pigtail catheters and can cause significant trauma during insertion, cause pain, prevent full lung expansion, and worsen pulmonary outcomes.[38] Pigtail catheters—smaller and less invasive than chest tubes—have been used successfully in patients with non-traumatic pneumothorax (e.g., those occurring during pacemaker implantation).

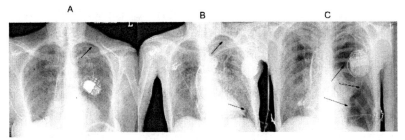

Figure 10. Examples of Pneumothoraces, Small (A), Medium (B), and Large (C). The edge of the pneumothorax is indicated by the arrows. A small left apical pneumothorax is shown in A. A moderate-sized apical and basilar pneumothorax is shown in B. An almost complete collapse of the left lung is shown in C. Please note that the examples shown in B and C are from defibrillator implantations. (Figure originally published by Williams and Stevenson[16])

Vascular access and bleeding (Hemothorax): The axillary venous approach has been associated with less frequent pneumothorax and subclavian crush syndrome (damage to the vein that can cause the arm to swell).[39,40] The axillary vein is the continuation of the basilica vein—it runs over the bicep muscle in the arm—that terminates immediately beneath the collar bone at the outer border of the first rib, at which point it becomes the subclavian vein.[41] Direct subclavian venous punctures are associated with increased rate of pneumothorax[37] while cephalic vein cut down has been associated with the lowest rate of pneumothorax and lead damage.[14,16]

Fluoroscopic-guided, first-rib approach to axillary vein access is the most effective means to access the vessel while minimizing the risk of pneumothorax.[41] The cephalic vein cut down is an advanced technique that allows us to place pacemakers' wires without poking a needle in the patient's chest wall; not all implanting physicians can perform this technique, so check with your implanting physician to see if this is an option.

Hemothorax (bleeding into the rib cage around the lungs) can be caused by pacemaker lead placement (more frequently atrial lead perforation) as well as vascular access damage to the subclavian and axillary veins and the vena cava. A prior study examined pacemaker implantation complication rates of 632 consecutive implants at a single non-community institution.[14] They found a 0.6% rate of hemothorax with a substantially large incidence of complications experienced by low-volume (fewer than twelve implants per year) implanters. **Figure 11** depicts a post-implant CXR of a hemothorax occurring during upgrade of dual-chamber pacemaker to biventricular defibrillator. Recognition of new effusions should be treated as possible procedural-related hemothorax, and surgical consultation is warranted.

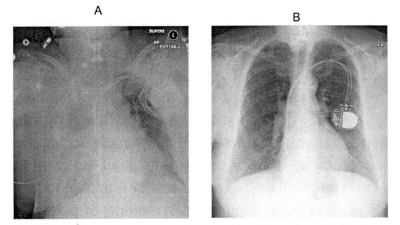

Figure 11. Hemothorax after Device Implantation. The right hemi-thorax has a layered effusion with blunting of the right diaphragm (hazy portion on left side of image A). Image B depicts the preoperative radiograph prior to upgrade of pacemaker to defibrillator. (Figure originally published by Williams and Stevenson[16])

It is important to ask your doctor the type of implant technique he or she uses. Again, an important question to ask is: How many devices has he or she implanted? No matter what vascular access technique used, generally, the more experience a doctor has, the lower the complication rate.

Perforation /Tamponade. Perforation occurs when trauma causes an unintended hole in a blood vessel or the walls of the heart; it can be a life-threatening situation. Perforation (both acute and subacute) has been reported to occur in up to 1% of pacemaker implantations.[16,19,27,28] In addition, asymptomatic subclinical (does not cause worrisome symptoms) perforation may occur in 15% of patients after device implantation.[42] Symptoms of perforation include: pleuritic chest pain from pericarditis, diaphragmatic or intercostal muscle stimulation (feel like involuntary and sometimes painful hiccups) and, in the presence of pericardial effusion (blood collecting around the outside of the heart), patients may develop shortness of breath and hypotension as tamponade develops.[43] Tamponade occurs when enough blood collects on the outside of the heart that it can compress the heart and render it unable to pump blood effectively. Other signs/symptoms of perforation include EKG abnormalities or friction rub (sounds like rubbing sandpaper heard on stethoscope) after implant. If perforation is suspected, urgent evaluation of the patient and device function is warranted, though lead parameters are often within normal limits.[43]

Figure 12 shows examples of coronary sinus damage that can occur during LV lead implantation (during defibrillator placements in these examples). **Figure 13** depicts right ventricular lead perforations. Cardiac surgery is typically not required for a majority of patients diagnosed with cardiac perforation from a pacemaker implantation. Rather, most cases can be managed with pericardiocentesis (drainage of blood with a small catheter) performed by an interventional cardiologist for symptomatic effusions and by repositioning of the lead in the EP laboratory with close cardiothoracic surgical collaboration.[43,44,45] **Figure 14** shows a large cardiac silhouette—developing after pacemaker implantation—that was due to large pericardial effusion. The effusion was treated with pericardiocentesis (with no evidence of blood re-accumulation) and did not require lead repositioning. Though perforation and subsequent tamponade are infrequent complications of pacemaker implantation, they can be responsible for significant patient morbidity and mortality. The risks of perforation cannot be underestimated; death from tamponade with subsequent cardiac arrest was responsible for 21.8% of the deaths in a worldwide study of perforation after ablation for atrial fibrillation.[46] There is some evidence that passive fixation leads cause fewer ventricular perforations, because there is no screw at the tip of the lead; indeed, most of my ventricular pacing leads are passive fixation, because I wish to avoid possibly catastrophic complications. The selection of passive versus active fixation involves many factors: such as patient anatomy, risk of complications, and implanter experience. It is important to ask your doctor what leads they will be using for your pacemaker—and why.

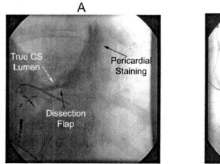

Figure 12. Damage to the coronary sinus during left ventricular lead implantation Image A depicts a dissection/perforation flap and the resulting pericardial staining from engaging the coronary sinus with a deflectable electrophysiology-recording catheter. Image B shows a similar instance of pericardial staining with no focal dissection flap or perforation. Both patients underwent successful LV lead implantation at the time. (Figure originally published by Williams and Stevenson[16])

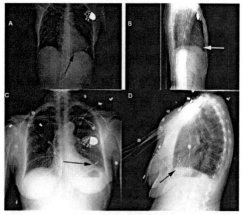

Figure 13. Examples of Right Ventricular Pacemaker Lead perforation. Images A and B depict an RV lead perforation that exits the right ventricular base in A (arrow) and reenters near the right ventricular apex in B (arrow). Images C and D depict a right ventricular apical perforation. The lead is seen exiting the cardiac silhouette in C (arrow); the lateral view (D) depicts an abrupt change in lead course (arrow) that is often seen in right ventricular apical perforations as the lead courses posteriorly in the pericardial space. (Figure originally published by Williams and Stevenson[16])

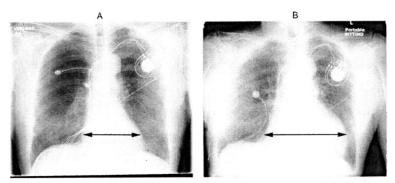

Figure 14. Chest radiograph appearance of large pericardial effusion after RV lead perforation. Immediate post-implant CXR (A) shows normal appearance of the cardiac silhouette. Two weeks post-operative CXR performed, because patient reported symptoms of chest pressure (B) shows enlarged cardiac silhouette. Patient responded to pericardiocentesis with no lead repositioning. (Figure originally published by Williams and Stevenson[16])

Complications of left ventricular (LV) lead placement via the coronary sinus. Resynchronization pacemakers are often used for patients with heart failure by placing a pacing lead in the left ventricle to "resynchronize" the pumping action of the heart so that the right and left ventricles pump at the same time. The emergence of resynchronization therapy has led to an increase in attempts at LV lead placement via the coronary sinus. The MIRACLE study program[47] reported a 91.6% success rate for LV lead placement, while COMPANION[48] revealed an 89% success rate for LV lead placement. Another report indicated a similar 92% success rate with LV lead placement.[49] Though I counsel my patients on an LV lead placement success rate at 88–92%, we have demonstrated a 97% success rate (sixty-four of sixty-six patients) with LV lead placement within the range from

2:30 to 5:30 o'clock in the left anterior oblique (LAO) view.[19]

Complications of biventricular pacing, specifically LV lead placement, include: cardiac perforation (poking hole in wall of vessel), coronary sinus dissection (damaging the vessel wall), electrical trauma (heart block), failure to place the lead, dislodgement of the lead, and diaphragmatic stimulation.[50] Coronary sinus dissections or perforations, cardiac perforations, or cardiac vein dissection or perforation were reported in forty-five of 2078 (2%) in the MIRACLE study program.[47] **Figure 12** depicts damage done to the coronary sinus during LV lead implantation. Loss of LV capture and diaphragmatic stimulation leading to interruption of resynchronization therapy have been found to occur in 10% and 2% of patients, respectively.[51] Diaphragmatic stimulation occurs when the pacing lead is placed too close to the phrenic nerve and can actually pace the diaphragm. This diaphragmatic pacing is not dangerous, though it can be uncomfortable; it feels like a "grabbing" or hiccup in the left chest or rib cage. The development of new LV leads with up to four electrodes (Quartet™, St. Jude Medical, Inc.) offers the possibility of numerous pacing locations that can minimize loss of capture and diaphragmatic stimulation.

Arrhythmias (supraventricular tachycardia, ventricular tachycardia, ventricular fibrillation) The incidence of sustained atrial, pacemaker-mediated, and ventricular rhythm disturbances after pacemaker implantation is low.[52] In patients without prior atrial arrhythmias, Jordaens et al found early atrial fibrillation (during the first week after implantation) in two of 112 patients, late atrial fibrillation was seen in seven patients, and atrial flutter was seen in one—yielding a total incidence of 8.9% for twenty-two months. There were no significant differences with respect to age, etiology (cause), electrocardiographic diagnosis, pacing history, or the measured intracardiac P wave between the group with and the group without atrial fibrillation. Ventricular fibrillation has been reported to occur in 0.1% of all patients undergoing pacemaker implantation and up to 0.6% of patients aged greater than ninety years undergoing pacemaker implantation.[16]

It has been reported that ventricular tachyarrhythmias (e.g., ventricular tachycardia or fibrillation) may be present in 12–31% of patients months to years after pacemaker implantation,[53] but this may reflect underlying progression of heart disease. However, there are several situations where pacemaker implantation may cause the ventricular tachyarrhythmias. These include: pacemaker lead irritation of the right ventricular inflow[54] and outflow tracts,[55] pacemaker stimulus on T wave,[56] reentrant circuit around endocardial pacemaker lead[57] and bradycardia-dependent VT facilitated by long pause caused by myopotential inhibition of a VVI pacemaker.[58]

Heart attacks. Heart attacks are also called myocardial infarctions (MI's) and are the most common cause of death after any surgery. This generally occurs in less than 1% of pacemaker surgeries. Again, the implanting physician generally assesses the risk of surgery prior to the procedure, and patients at high risk of heart attacks may need additional heart care prior to proceeding with pacemaker implantation.

Death. In-hospital death generally occurs in less than 1% of pacemaker implantations;[16,28] however, there is a concern that death is underreported, because some studies do not specifically mention perioperative death.[14,16] The most common causes of confirmed device-related in-hospital deaths are perforations of the subclavian artery, brachiocephalic trunk, right atrium, and right ventricle. The most common cause of non-device related in-hospital deaths is myocardial infarction (heart attack) as well as, less commonly, pulmonary embolism, stroke, heart failure, and sepsis.[59]

Pocket hematoma. A pocket hematoma is a collection of blood around the pacemaker device but underneath the skin. **Figure 15F** shows an example of a pocket hematoma. The incidence of pocket hematoma has been reported at 4.9% and leading to prolonged hospitalization in 2.0% of all patients.[60] Reoperation for pocket hematoma—to drain the collection of blood—may occur in up to 1.0% of patients. High-dose heparinization, combined acetylsalicylic acid (ASA or aspirin)/thienopyridine (such as clopidogrel, Plavix®) treatment after coronary stenting, and low operator experience were independently predictive of hematoma development.[60] In addition, development of postoperative hematoma places the patient at elevated risk of device infection.[61] Most hematomas resolve with watchful waiting and do not require a repeat surgery. They resolve over four to six weeks and can often have significant associated bruising, which also resolves over that time period. Worrisome signs include: continued swelling, redness, warmth, bleeding, oozing, or changes in the incision. It is important to call the implanting physician with any worries about incision or pocket healing.

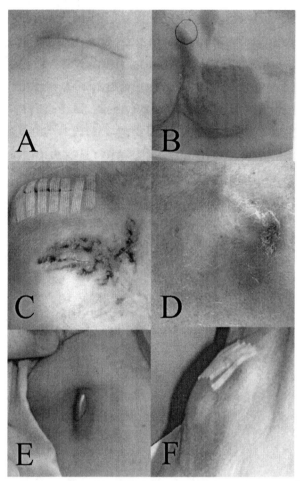

Figure 15A-F. Examples of Incisional Healing Normal pacemaker pocket (A) several weeks after implantation shows a uniform incision and mild fullness representing the pacemaker in the pocket. Pocket and incisional thinning with prominent skin tenting from a lead (circle) in an extremely elderly patient is shown in B. Redness and irritation from adhesive tape is shown in C. One can see redness and skin breakdown that is seen with imminent erosion (D) than can lead to complete erosion (breaks through the skin) of pacemaker (E). Finally, F depicts a pocket hematoma.

There is data to suggest that warfarin (Coumadin®) causes fewer pocket complications than heparin products. Specifically, temporarily interrupting anticoagulation (e.g., stopping Coumadin) is associated with increased thromboembolic events (e.g., strokes or transient ischemic attacks), whereas cessation of warfarin with bridging anticoagulation with heparin products is associated with a higher rate of pocket hematoma and a longer hospital stay.[62] The discussion of perioperative anticoagulation is very important to discuss with the doctor who will be performing the pacemaker implantation.

Hospital lengths of stay: There is little data available on average length of hospital stays post pacemaker implantation. Our experience with pacemaker implantation in extremely elderly patients[84] revealed an average hospital length of stay post-implant of 2.1 days; however, over 90% of pacemaker generator changes were discharged home the same day, and most patients that had an elective pacemaker implant (e.g., referred from the office) were discharged the day after implantation. An estimate of two to three days as an average length of stay post implant can be made from the available studies, though this includes patients that were already admitted to the hospital for other reasons.[16,19,84] There is evidence that complications cause a substantial increase in the length of stay up to sixteen days.63 The mean complication costs are: $4345 ± $1540 for pacemaker lead revision, $24,459 ± $14,585 for pacemaker infection, and $6187 ± $2631 for hematoma evacuation.[63]

Complications that usually occur within thirty days of implant.

Pacemaker and lead function/failures: Electrocardio-graphic signs of pacemaker malfunction can be grouped into four categories: failure to pace the heart, failure to deliver a pacing signal, undersensing, and inappropriate pacemaker rate. There is an overall pacemaker and lead malfunction rate in 1–3% of patients.[64]

Failure to pace the heart (loss of capture). Failure to pace the heart means that a pacing signal is delivered but does not result in a heartbeat. You may not even notice this occurring, but patients can often feel palpitations or dizziness or even faint as a result. Loss of capture after pacemaker implantation has many causes:

- *Dislodgement*. Lead dislodgement means that the lead has fallen out of place and likely is in an area that does not pace correctly.

- *Elevated thresholds*: Device requires more energy than normal to pace and may lead to early battery depletion.

- *Inappropriate lead placement*: Lead may not be properly located and misplacement not discovered until follow-up.

- *Lead fracture*: Very rarely a lead may break (usually near insertion site to pacemaker header).

- *Insulation failure*: The silicone/plastic outer coating of the lead (insulator) has a defect and can cause lead to malfunction.

- *Loose set screw*: The screw that holds lead in the pacemaker header may become loose.

- *Exit block (greater than four weeks)*: Scar formation developing at the tip of the lead where it contacts the heart makes pacing more difficult.

- *Perforation*: The leads poke through the wall of the heart and may lead to bleeding or more serious complications.

- *Battery/circuit failure*: Very rare and discussed in **chapter ten**.

- *Air in pocket*: During surgery, some air may remain in pocket and at times can cause issues until the air reabsorbs over several weeks.

- *Metabolic/Drugs (Flecainide)*: Medications and some illnesses can make it difficult for the lead to pace the heart.

Lead dislodgement, the most common cause of failure to capture,[64] has been reported to occur in up to 4–6% of pacemaker implantations but is generally reported with a 1–3% incidence.[16,19,27,28] **Figures 16 and 17** depict examples of right atrial, right ventricular, and left ventricular lead dislodgements that may result in failure to pace the heart. Lead dislodgements are treated by repositioning the lead in the implant procedure room.

A. Initial Post-Implant CXR   B. CXR After "Twiddling"

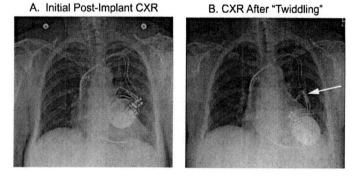

Figure 16. Lead orientation before and after patient twiddling resulted in lead dislodgement. Twiddling refers to patient manipulation of pacemaker can or leads that may lead to malfunction. Image A depicts the post-implant radiograph baseline lead positioning after biventricular defibrillator implant. Image B shows retracted right and left ventricular leads and leads tangled in the pocket superior to device can that is rotated. (Figure originally published by Williams and Stevenson[16])

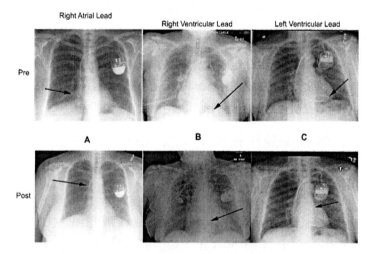

Figure 17. Right Atrial (A), Right Ventricular (B), and Left Ventricular (C) Leads Before (Pre) and After (Post) Dislodgements. Right atrial lead became dislodged after patient twiddled with device. Right ventricular lead dislodged by moving more basilar in position (arrow) one day after implant. Left ventricular lead dislodged and reseated itself in the body of coronary sinus three months after initial placement (arrow). (Figure originally published by Williams and Stevenson[16])

Failure to output: Failure of the device to deliver a pacemaker signal may be caused by: battery or circuit failure, lead fracture, internal insulation failure, oversensing, loose set screw, or crosstalk. Complete pacemaker failure (due to a random component failure) is quite rare; however, total battery depletion can occur if routine pacemaker follow-up is inadequate.[64] Once initial end-of-life indicators appear, there is usually a period of months before the battery reaches a critically low voltage and pacing fails.[64] The incidence of pacemaker lead fracture (e.g., the lead breaks) has been reported at 0.1–4.2% per patient-year and usually occurs adjacent to the generator or near the site of venous access.[65] Other electrical signals may cause noise and subsequent "oversensing" (and fool the pacemaker into not pacing); most commonly, the diaphragm's contracting can cause electrical signals (myopotentials) to be detected by the pacemaker (oversensing) and misinterpreted by the pacemaker as normal heartbeats (and the pacemaker will stop pacing). Also, other sources of external electrical noise can affect pacing function (discussed in **chapter eight**).

Undersensing: Undersensing of intrinsic heartbeats results in inappropriate pacing output that competes with your native heartbeat. Undersensing is most likely caused by lead dislodgement, poor lead position at time of implantation, or an interruption in the insulation of the pacing lead.[64]

Inappropriate pacemaker rate: There are several causes of inappropriate pacemaker rate but most are not due to device malfunction except "runaway pacemaker." A runaway pacemaker" is a true device failure that can rarely be caused by battery depletion, random component failure, or radiation treatments for cancer.[64] The more common causes of inappropriate pacemaker rate are not actual malfunctions of the pacemaker but issues that can be corrected by altering the pacemaker's programming. Pacing can be too slow if the device is oversensing or too fast if the device is undersensing. See above for descriptions of oversensing and undersensing.

Hospital readmission: The average rate of hospital readmission within thirty days of pacemaker implant is 4–6%.[16,19,84] There are many factors that can increase the likelihood of readmission to the hospital after a pacemaker implantation. Increased age and increased device complexity (e.g., generator changes that do not involve placement of new pacemaker leads are less complex than devices that require multiple new lead placements) may increase readmission rate.[16,84] Other factors that can increase risk of readmission include: abnormal kidney function, emergency situation/presentation, ejection fraction, female gender, and small stature (weight less than one hundred pounds). Reasons for readmission are quite varied, but many result from the aforementioned complications in addition to: heart failure, pneumonia, or strokes. Of note, the vast majority of patients that require pacemakers is aged greater than sixty-five years and often has other medical conditions that may be exacerbated by any surgical procedure.

Strokes: Strokes (also called transient ischemic attacks or TIAs) may occur immediately postoperatively or can occur several weeks out from implantation. Strokes generally occur in less than 1% of patients but have been seen in up to 1.4% of extremely elderly (age greater than eighty years) patients undergoing pacemaker implantation.[84] I have most commonly seen strokes in patients that had anticoagulation (warfarin or Coumadin©) held temporarily for the surgery; the strokes occur during the time the anticoagulation was held until the patient has been effectively reanticoagulated after the surgery. There is data to suggest that pacemaker implantation can be safely performed without stopping warfarin and may lead to fewer complications.[62] It is important to discuss management of anticoagulants with the implanting physician prior to surgery.

Death (also called mortality) is unusual after pacemaker implantation, though it is a risk of any procedure. Early all-cause mortality, thirty days after pacemaker implantation, has been reported in 0.1–0.7% of patients.[16] Death rates may be increased (2%) in the extreme elderly aged greater than eighty years due to increased age-related mortality in this group.[84]

Complications that usually occur more than one month after implant.

Lead function/Failures: Twiddling: Originally described in 1968,[66] twiddling refers to patient manipulation of the pacemaker can or leads that may result in malfunction. It has a reported incidence of 0.07% in a series of seventeen thousand patients.[67] **Figure 16** depicts lead orientation before and after patient twiddling resulted in lead dislodgement. *Exit block*: Sometimes pacemaker leads require more voltage than normal to adequately pace the heart. Transient disruptions to pacing function can be caused by; systemic disease states (like infection) and electrolyte abnormalities, drug effects, extreme hypothyroidism (low thyroid), and coronary artery disease (cardiac ischemia). There is an expected rise in voltage requirements in the two to six week period after lead placement attributed to local inflammation or foreign-body reaction at the tip-tissue interface. The degree that the capture threshold increases is markedly blunted with steroid-eluting pacemaker leads, which have thus become generally preferred for their more favorable delivery characteristics, having overcome the problem of higher stimulation thresholds.[68,69]

Of note, most current pacing leads are active fixation (meaning the lead is actively fixed to the heart by a corkscrew-like helix at the tip). These active fixation leads tend to have a slightly higher pacing requirement. Passive fixation leads (see **chapter four**) have a capture threshold relatively lower than standard active fixation leads. The disadvantages to passive fixation leads are an inability to perform atrial mapping, unreliable lateral wall stability, and requirement for placement in the atrial appendage—which may be difficult in patients who have undergone bypass. A rise in capture threshold may occur beyond six weeks after implantation: the chronic phase of lead maturation. As the threshold steadily rises, it may exceed the maximum output of the pulse generator, known as *exit block*. Exit block is recognized by high pacing thresholds without radiographic evidence of dislodgement. It may be related to inflammation or fibrosis at the electrode-myocardium interface and generally presents greater than four weeks after implantation.[64] Some patients—particularly pediatric patients—are particularly prone to this phenomenon, and it may require multiple lead revisions.

Device/Lead advisories. See **chapter ten.**

Infection. Infection is estimated to occur in 0.5-2% of patients. Of these infections, up to 60% of patients present with localized infection involving the device pocket, whereas the remaining patients may present with endovascular infection but no evidence of inflammation of the device pocket.[17] Approximately 10% of patients may have intracardiac vegetations identified by transesophageal echocardiogram, though they can still undergo percutaneous lead extraction safely.[70] The risk of pacemaker infection is lower than that of implantable defibrillators. The presence of epicardial leads (placed during heart surgery) and postoperative complications at the generator pocket (e.g., pocket hematoma) are significant risk factors for early-onset device infection, whereas longer duration of hospitalization at the time of implantation and chronic obstructive pulmonary disease were associated with late-onset device infections.[16] In one of the largest studies of pacemaker infections,[71] repeated operative procedures after the first pacemaker implantation were associated with a substantial incremental risk of infection. Female gender, older age, and preoperative antibiotics given at the initial implant were associated with a lower risk of later infection. The pacing mode, indication for pacing, and complexity of the procedure were not independently associated with the risk of later infection. Sixty percent of infections have been found to occur within ninety days of implant,[72] though a large number of infections occur during the late stage (greater than one year post-implant).[71] Generator changes and cardiac resynchronization therapy/dual-chamber devices have also been implicated as independent predictors of infection.[72]

The generally accepted means of device infection treatment is removal of the generator and all implanted leads.[2] In a large series of device extractions, including 1,838 leads,[70] post-operative thirty-day mortality was 10%, though no deaths were related directly to the extraction procedure. Another series of device extractions reported: a 0.5% rate of intraprocedural mortality, a 4.6% rate of in-hospital mortality, and a 2.6% rate of relapsing infections within one year of reimplantation.[17]

Device infection is a very serious complication, and any worrisome symptoms—such as fever, chills, redness, or drainage of the incision—should be reported to your doctor.

Pacemaker syndrome. This syndrome occurs most commonly with single-chamber ventricular pacemakers (e.g., VVI or VVIR modes). Symptoms are due to loss of atrioventricular (AV) synchrony. The loss of AV synchrony means that the top chambers of your heart (the atria) may be pumping against contracting bottom chambers (the ventricles) and lead to uncomfortable symptoms. It must be noted that pacemaker syndrome can occur with any pacing mode if AV synchrony is lost. Symptoms include: malaise, weakness, chest pain, cough, confusion, or syncope (fainting).

Venous thrombosis. Upper-extremity deep-venous thrombosis (or stenosis) is uncommon in the general population, but venous stenosis has been seen in up to 33–64% of patients after implantation of pacing leads.[73,74] Statistically significant factors that have been associated with an increased risk include: previous transvenous temporary leads,[74] left ventricular ejection fraction less than 40%,[74] systemic infection,[75] absence of anticoagulation, use of hormone treatment, personal history of venous thrombosis, and presence of multiple leads.[76] Symptoms may include: shoulder or neck discomfort, ipsilateral (same side as pacemaker) arm swelling with cyanosis (bluish discoloration), dilated collateral cutaneous veins around the shoulder, or jugular vein distension.[77] Venography is considered the gold standard for diagnosis, but compressive ultrasonography is an effective and economical means of confirming the clinical diagnosis.[77] Treatment may include: anticoagulation (warfarin and/or heparin), extraction of the old nonfunctioning lead to create a new venous channel, or venoplasty to reduce venous stenosis or allow the implantation of subsequent leads.[77,78]

CHAPTER 8
Post-Operative Care (The First Month):

Each implanting physician and practice will have slightly different post-operative care instructions, and it is important to check with your doctor regarding special instructions after pacemaker implantation. I will be summarizing the limitations/restrictions I recommend to patients following pacemaker implantation. You should confirm activity limitations/restrictions with your own doctor.

Care of the incision (showering/bathing). Proper healing of the incision is critical to avoid infections after the implantation. For this reason, I recommend no tub baths or showers for seven days after the implantation—the average duration of restriction ranges from two to fourteen days. The patient should not get water, soap, ointments, or salves on or near the incision during this time (unless instructed by the implanting physician). Once the incision has healed during this initial period, the patient can begin showering, and any superficial bandages (e.g., Steri-Strips®) will begin to fall off on their own. I use three layers of absorbable sutures (stitches) to close the incision, and these will slowly get absorbed by the body during the normal healing process. Some doctors use staples to close the skin layer of a pacemaker incision; the patient will have to return to the doctor's office in one to two weeks to remove the staples. The same bathing instructions apply to patients with staples in place.

It is normal for the incision to be sore after device implantation. There will be mild tenderness at the incision site that should be improving on a daily basis. If the pain is getting worse or the incision gets redder or more swollen or feels hot, the patient should call the implanting physician. The vast majority of my patients require only non-narcotic pain relief (e.g., Advil® or Tylenol®) after the implantation, but some patients may require a few days of narcotic pain relief after the implantation.

The incision itself may look slightly red for the first several days, but each day it should get less and less red. If there is any increasing redness, warmth, or swelling, the implanting physician should be notified. You may see some dried blood along the incision, and this can be normal; if bleeding persists or the incision continues to ooze or leak fluid, the implanting physician should be notified. **Figure 15** depicts examples of both normal (**figure 15A**) and abnormal incisions and pacemaker pockets (**figure 15C–F**). You can typically see (and feel) the outline of the pacemaker and mild soft tissue swelling in a pocket that is healing normally. There should be no significant tension on the incision; the incision should not look like it is being "stretched" because of swelling underneath. A pocket hematoma is an abnormal collection of blood around the device, but underneath the incision, that looks like swelling. You can see exaggerated fullness around a pacemaker with a hematoma present (**Figure 15F**) not seen in a normally healing pacemaker site. Finally, some thin patients may only have a very thin layer of skin over the healed pacemaker site (**Figure 15B**), and you may even see the course of the pacemaker lead. As long as there is no abnormal redness or tenderness, this can be a normal finding. Again, any concern about the incision healing should be relayed to your doctor.

Symptoms that should be reported immediately to a physician:

- Fevers or chills
- Incisional redness, warmth, tenderness, or swelling
- Drainage or bleeding from the incision site
- Chest pain, shortness of breath, difficulty breathing
- Hiccups or abnormal "twitching" of chest wall or ribcage muscles
- Swelling in arms, wrists, legs, or ankles
- Fainting (syncope), lightheadedness, or dizziness
- Palpitations or fast, racing heartbeat
- Severe weakness or fatigue
- Any dramatic change or development of symptoms immediately following the implant

Activity limitations. Patients should not raise the implant-side arm above shoulder height or behind their back for four weeks after the implantation. In addition, I recommend that patients not lift more than five pounds (or a gallon of milk) during these four weeks. These restrictions give the pacemaker leads a chance to scar in place. It must be noted that it can take up to six weeks for the leads to become securely anchored in the pocket. In addition, it may take several months for the leads to become scarred in place in the heart. Any sudden trauma (such as a fall or car accident) within the first several months after implantation can lead to pacemaker lead dislodgement. Contact sports and vigorous activity should be avoided during these first four weeks. Of note, I generally recommend that contact sports (e.g., football and rugby) and vigorous activity that involves significant jarring (e.g., horseback riding) be avoided in any patients that have a pacemaker. You should ask your doctor about any activity that may involve excessive jarring or trauma.

Driving. I generally recommend that patients not drive until the first follow-up appointment: ten to fourteen days after implantation. This allows me to make sure the incision is healing properly and leads are functioning appropriately. Obviously, if the patient experiences any alterations in consciousness—when a person faints, we call it syncope—prior to receiving the pacemaker implantation, the patient should not drive until their physician deems it safe to drive. Each state is different, but Pennsylvania law suggests that patients should not drive for six months if the reason for their syncope can be fully explained and they have no further episodes of syncope during this time. It is recommended that the patient not drive for twelve months from the last episode of fainting (syncope) if no cause is identified. Please check with your doctor prior to resuming driving.

The first follow-up appointment after the pacemaker implantation. The patient usually receives a card describing the maker of the device and leads; this is important information to know in case of an emergency. A follow-up visit is usually arranged for one to two weeks from the device implant. I have the patient return for a visit with our pacemaker clinic to assess the incision, check the device, and continue the pacemaker education process. Some patients are required to follow-up with separate doctors for the incision check (if surgeon implanted device) and device check (performed at the cardiologist's or primary care provider's office). After this initial visit, the patient will be scheduled for an in-office device evaluation and ongoing education at three months post-implant. These evaluations may occur over the phone (transtelephonic monitoring) or in person if the device cannot be remotely monitored. Each physician offers different follow-up options. Most of the new devices offer remote monitoring via a secure website. This allows the patient to have their device checked from home. This remote monitoring is especially convenient for patients with limited mobility or transportation options. These visits/checks allow your doctor to make sure the device and leads are working appropriately and the battery is okay. Moreover, remote monitoring can allow your doctor to track your heart failure and detect arrhythmias, such as atrial fibrillation.

Lifestyle considerations. One of the major concerns is that a pacemaker will dramatically affect the patient's lifestyle. Once the temporary activity limitations are lifted (generally at four weeks), there are very few changes that need to be made to one's lifestyle. First, most home electronic devices are safe for use with a pacemaker. Any properly grounded, handheld electronic device is safe as long as it is kept a safe distance from the pacemaker site—approximately six inches is a good rule of thumb. Microwave ovens are safe to use (and I jokingly tell patients "as long as you don't climb inside!"). Induction ovens may emit noise that can interfere with a pacemaker, and you should stay several feet away from a working induction oven. Any device that has electrical output could cause pacemaker malfunction. The most common malfunction is that the interfering device causes the pacemaker to "oversense" noise and fool the pacemaker into stopping pacing. I have seen this happen with transcutaneous electrical nerve stimulators (TENS units). Another malfunction I have seen involves improper household grounding. During flooding in our region, a pacemaker patient went into a flooded basement, and the device inappropriately recognized external noise (from a shorted furnace) as normal heart electrical activity and stopped pacing. Most home power tools are safe to use when kept at arms' length; however, gas-powered tools (especially chain saws) may cause interference with the pacemaker. Check with your doctor prior to using any gas-powered tools.

I do not recommend that patients linger in or near the security exit for stores; there is a slim chance of electrical noise from these areas. There are several situations that can interfere with pacemaker operation, and **table 4** lists many procedures that may interfere with your pacemaker. Arc welding produces large amounts of electrical noise, and you cannot expose a pacemaker to these fields. This electrical noise can cause your pacemaker to stop pacing or pace at the wrong time. If you think an electric field is affecting pacemaker function, you should move away from the source of the noise. Any powerful electrical or magnetic field can interfere with a pacemaker. Companies are developing MRI-approved pacemakers (Revo MRI Surescan Pacing System, Medtronic, Inc.) that may safely allow a patient to undergo an MRI scan. Interestingly, there are some centers that will allow patients with pacemakers to undergo MRI scanning, but every center is different. Please check with your doctor about MRI scanning and if you will require MRI scans. Your doctor may consider an MRI-approved pacemaker system.

I advise patients to avoid any activity that involves rough physical contact. Strenuous activities such as basketball, football, tennis, or racquetball could cause jarring and damage to the pacemaker or leads. In addition, you would not want to use a rifle on the same side as your pacemaker. Finally, if you are unsure if an activity/environment is safe for a pacemaker, please check with your doctor.

Table 4. Procedures that may Interfere with Pacemaker Function. This table describes many procedures that pacemaker patients undergo. These are meant as general guidelines. Always discuss the safety of any procedure with your doctor if you have a pacemaker.

SAFE	LOW RISK	MEDIUM/ HIGH RISK	UNSAFE
Dental procedures	CAT Scans	Electrocautery	MRI
X-rays	Ventilators (Breathing machines)	Hearing aids with coil around neck	Diathermy (Tissue heating that may be used by chiropractor)
In-ear hearing aids	Ultrasound	Tissue ablation	
Mammography	Electrolysis	Lithotripsy	
		Radiation therapy	
		TENS units	

CHAPTER 9
Long-Term Care and Follow-Up:

Follow-up. As described in **chapter eight**, patients will have regularly scheduled pacemaker evaluations every three to twelve months. These evaluations may be performed in the office or performed remotely (from the patient's home). The pacemaker programming, lead function, and battery strength are routinely checked as well as any malfunction or manufacturer alert (see **chapter ten** to learn about recalls/advisories). Many practices (including mine) schedule remote monitoring on a three-month basis to follow patients closely for possible lead malfunction, battery life, and any other additional alerts the pacemaker has been programmed to monitor. Newer devices offer the ability for pacemakers to track the patient's weight (requires a scale designed for that device), volume status (by measuring chest-wall impedance), and respiratory rate. These parameters can help your doctor monitor for heart failure.

Pacemaker function: During a routine pacemaker inter-rogation (remotely or in the office, see **figure 7**), your pacemaker function will be evaluated in a systematic way. First, the pacemaker clinic staff will place the wand over the pacemaker site—some newer devices are fully wireless—and download a current status update for the pacemaker. This initial report will reveal any alerts/warnings that occurred since the last check as well as parameters that help us determine the remaining battery life and lead functions. The leads are evaluated based upon three main characteristics: (1) amplitude, (2) threshold, and (3) impedance.

> *Amplitude*: This refers to the voltage that your heart creates during a normal heartbeat. The size (or amplitude) of this voltage helps us determine how to program your device as well as how the lead is functioning. If the amplitude becomes too small, the pacemaker may not be able to detect your native heartbeat. If the device cannot sense your native heartbeat (called undersensing), it may pace excessively.

> *Threshold*: This refers to how much energy (volt-age and current) is required to cause your heart to beat (we call this capture). The lower the thresh-old, the less energy required to pace your heart and the longer the battery life.

Impedance: Impedance is a measure of the opposition in current that is present in the pacemaker lead. In other words, a normally functioning pacemaker lead has a certain range of normal impedance. An abnormal drop in this impedance may represent breakdown of the insulating material of the lead. An abnormal increase in impedance may represent a defect in the pacemaker's wires.

Patient monitoring features of pacemakers

Arrhythmia burden: Most pacemakers have the ability to detect and record any occurrences of arrhythmias: such as atrial fibrillation or ventricular tachycardia. Often, the first time atrial fibrillation is detected is from the pacemaker's alerts.

Hemodynamic monitoring: Many pacemakers have the ability to monitor daily patient activity, volume status (via thoracic impedance), heart rates, and respiratory rates. The ability to track hemodynamic parameters like this permits us to make adjustments to medications.

Lead/Device advisories: Most pacemakers have alarms programmed that will alert us to possible lead or device problems: such as lead damage, battery/circuit failure, or software malfunctions. These alerts are reviewed during pacemaker checks.

Incision care. Generally, incisions have mostly healed four to six weeks after the pacemaker implantation, but it is important to routinely check your incision. Scarring can be minimized by applying sunscreen over the healed incision; check with your physician when it is safe to apply sunscreen to your incision. Any cracking, oozing, bleeding, swelling, or redness should be reported immediately to your physician. Protect your incision and device pocket from any direct trauma or abrasion—from seatbelts in particular. Any device trauma should be reported to your physician, and device check should be performed remotely or in the office (to permit an examination of the incision and device pocket).

If your car's shoulder seatbelt crosses directly over where your device sits, it is worthwhile to use a sheepskin seatbelt cover to prevent *pocket erosion*. Pocket erosion is caused by thinning of the skin and tissue overlying the pacemaker (**figure 15B**) that can ultimately lead to skin breakdown (**figure 15D**), exposes the pacemaker, and leads to bacteria from the skin's surface. Pocket erosions (**figure 15E**) generally mandate complete device (and lead) removal (called extraction). Pacemaker extractions can be very dangerous and risky to the patient.

Finally, the patient should never manipulate (called *twiddling*) the device or leads. Patients that twiddle the pacemaker (e.g., rolling it over or sliding it side to side) can damage the leads and/or pacemaker. **Figure 16** shows retracted right and left ventricular leads and leads tangled in the pocket superior to a pacemaker can that has been rotated by twiddling. Leads may become dislodged and malfunction—requiring reoperation.

Battery/Lead life. The battery of a pacemaker is sealed within the metal can that includes the pacemaker circuitry. When the battery is depleted, the entire pacemaker is replaced. This involves opening the prior incision, disconnecting the existing leads, and attaching a new pacemaker to these leads. This procedure can usually be done as an outpatient, with the patient returning home later in the day. I generally have patients continue all their medications (including anticoagulation with warfarin), but check with your physician regarding medication regimen.

Pacemaker batteries generally last from five to eight years—depending on how much pacing the patient requires. I have had pacemakers last fifteen to twenty years if the patient is rarely being paced. Unless there is an advisory, alert, or recall (discussed in **chapter ten**), pacemaker batteries slowly run out, and depletion can be detected during routine device checks. Once the pacemaker reaches the Elective Replacement Indicator (ERI), it will generally continue to function for three to six months—allowing time to schedule the generator replacement procedure.

Pacemaker leads can have a variable life span. Often, the leads outlast the pacemaker itself and are reused with the new pacemaker during a pacemaker generator replacement. Prior to any pacemaker replacement, the leads are reevaluated to be sure they function properly and to determine if there are any recalls/advisories/alerts that may cause malfunction.

Traveling. It is okay to travel by air and go through security checkpoints with a pacemaker, though I recommend patients do not walk through the security's metal detector. I recommend they show their pacemaker ID card to security and have them "wand check" for metal objects. Routine pacemaker follow-up visits are very important, so if you plan to be away from home for several weeks to months, ask your physician to help find a physician at your travel destination that is available for unexpected health issues. Most pacemaker companies have an international presence for emergency device checks, but discuss international travel plans with your doctor and find out about any heart centers that are near your destination.

Can a pacemaker cause heart failure? Yes, but it is not common. Usually a person's heart has electrical activation from top to bottom. When a person is dependent on a pacemaker, the very tip of the bottom right chamber (right ventricle) is paced first; this causes the heart muscle to be activated in an unnatural sequence (called dyssynchrony). There have been studies that confirm pacing can cause mild heart failure as seen by an approximate 11% drop in ejection fraction.[79] Many patients may not notice this decrease in heart pumping function. However, patients at risk of heart failure after a pacemaker may benefit from a resynchronization pacemaker by having an additional lead placed in the left ventricle (biventricular pacing). This type of pacemaker consists of three leads: leads in the right atrium, right ventricle, and the extra lead in the left ventricle (placed via the coronary sinus). This special type of pacemaker has been demonstrated to prevent pacemaker-induced heart failure.[80] You should talk to your doctor to see if this is an appropriate option for you. Not all patients need this special type of pacemaker.

Do pacemakers keep extremely elderly patients alive and prevent natural death? No. Pacemakers do not keep terminally ill patients alive. Most events that cause death at end of life are due to things like: overwhelming infection (sepsis), bleeding, cancer, strokes, or major organ failure (kidney or liver). During these types of catastrophic events, the heart is too sick to be paced by the pacemaker. The current ACC/AHA/HRS Guidelines on Device Therapy state: "Clinicians should encourage patients undergoing device implantation to complete advanced directives and specifically address the matter of device management and deactivation if the patient is terminally ill."[81]

In cases where the patient, family, and/or clinician feel that the pacemaker is not providing the appropriate therapy/care (e.g., patients with severe, debilitating dementia), deactivation of the pacemaker is an option. It must be noted that many patients are not dependent upon the pacemaker, and it is rare that deactivation results in immediate patient death. Often, when death

CHAPTER 10
What are Device Recalls/ Advisories/Alerts?

Any time a pacemaker or lead may have a problem, that item is placed under *advisory*. This term is used rather than "recall," because the pacemaker or lead may have a small chance of failure. But for most patients, watchful waiting is the most appropriate option. Indeed, if a pacemaker or lead has to be replaced, the patient is subject to many of the same risks of the initial pacemaker implantation. A large multicenter Canadian observational study showed that the complication rate from device replacement for an advisory indication was an astounding 9.1%.[82] Of these, 5.9% required reoperation, and there were two deaths. Naturally, the risk of an adverse outcome during replacement must be balanced by the risk of death due to device malfunction. Pacemakers and defibrillators have saved thousands of lives, but as is true of all man-made devices, malfunctions will continue to occur.

In response to a marked increase in device advisories in 2005—and to balance alarmism with protection of patients with a high-risk situation—the Heart Rhythm Society (HRS) published guidelines in 2006 to aid physicians.[83] Recognizing that physicians and patients need timely and accurate information regarding device performance, arguably the most important outcome was a call for greater transparency of problems that occur with pacemakers that are currently in use and the reporting of failures. Device performance depends not only on the characteristics of the device but the skill of the implanting physician and caregivers following the device.[83] Using data compiled from 1990–2002, FDA annual reports showed that confirmed device malfunctions leading to device explantation were about 0.1–0.9% for pacemakers.[83] Although failure rates are low, there is a negative psychological impact on patients who have a device that is under advisory—particularly if they are pacemaker dependent.

To assist in communication from industry to physicians and patients, it was proposed that terminology be standardized. The term "recall" was changed to "Class I Advisory," which is just short of a recommendation for device replacement because of a reasonable probability that malfunction could result in death or significant harm. Class II and Class III recalls are subsequently referred to as advisory notices (non-life threatening malfunctions) and safety alerts (potential malfunctions). This information is disseminated from industry via standardized letters to physicians and patients; these letters are also available on the pacemaker manufacturer's website. Prior experience tells us the advisory information should be disseminated to physicians just before patients. Advisories should include general information about the malfunction and potential clinical implications but should acknowledge that treatment decisions should ultimately be determined by patients in consultations with physicians.

The situations where device replacement is recommended are: (1) when mechanism of malfunction is known and is likely to be recurrent or lead to patient death, (2) the patient is pacemaker dependent, (3) the device was placed for a secondary prevention indication or has received appropriate therapy, or (4) the device is approaching EOL. Conservative management (enhanced non-invasive and remote monitoring) should be considered when: (1) The rate of malfunction is very low in non-pacemaker-dependent patients, (2) the patient has significant comorbidities or high operative risk even when the risk of device malfunction is substantial, or (3) remote monitoring and software reprogramming can minimize risk (i.e., non-physiologic noise).

If you are concerned about a potential advisory for your pacemaker (or leads), contact your doctor. Of note: I often "mix and match" leads and pacemakers, so your

CHAPTER 11
Conclusion:

The elderly are the fastest growing segment of the US population, and they commonly undergo pacemaker implantation. Doctors' offices have short pamphlets about pacemaker implantation, but I've attempted to provide a comprehensive reference available for these patients and their families that explains the "what, why, and how" of pacemaker implantation.

This book provides an in-depth summary of pacemakers from initial patient evaluation and device implantation and the issues that may arise during long-term follow-up. The majority of the book is designed to educate patients that have or are under evaluation for a pacemaker. The section on complications is a useful review that is slanted toward a primary care provider's knowledge base; moreover, the book summarizes the most important issues that pacemaker patients and their families encounter once the pacemaker implantation is completed.

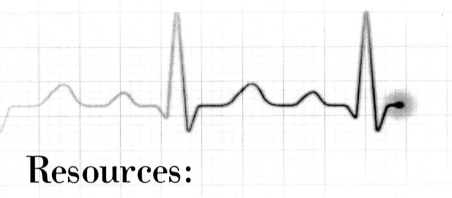

Resources:

Heart.org: This is the website for the American Heart Association. You will find exhaustive resources for physicians and patients about cardiovascular disease and stroke. Fellows of the American Heart Association (denoted by FAHA after his or her name) recognizes that particular physician's scientific and professional accomplishments and volunteer leadership and service dedicated to cardiovascular medicine.

Cardiosmart.org: This is the website for the American College of Cardiology. There is extensive information about cardiology for the patient and provider. Fellows of the American College of Cardiology (denoted by FACC after their name) are selected based on their outstanding credentials, achievements, and community contribution to promote excellence in cardiovascular care.

Hrsonline.org: The Heart Rhythm Society (HRS) is a leading resource on cardiac pacing and electrophysiology.

This specialty organization represents medical, allied health, and science professionals from more than seventy countries that specialize in cardiac rhythm disorders. HRS delivers programs and services to its membership. Fellows of the Heart Rhythm Society (denoted by FHRS after their name) have advanced training, certification, and demonstrated commitment to the research and treatment of heart rhythm disorders.

Heart-rhythm-center.com: This is Dr. Williams' discussion forum for biotechnology, pacemakers, defibrillators, and electrophysiology studies—including ablation. Patients and physicians can learn about and comment on a host of heart-rhythm-related topics.

Whatisapacemaker.com: This website serves as a discussion forum for readers of this book. Many aspects of the book are discussed, and readers are encouraged to give feedback and recommendations for topics in future editions.

Pacemaker Manufacturer Websites: The following is a list of the most commonly implanted pacemakers and their websites. They often have patient and physician educational resources that are very informative:

1. Biotronik: www.biotronik.com

2. Boston Scientific Corporation: www.bostonscientific.com

3. Medtronic, Inc.: www.medtronic.com

4. Soren Group USA, Inc.: www.soren.com

5. St. Jude Medical, Inc.: www.sjm.com

Glossary:

<u>Ablation:</u> Catheter-based electrical heating of tissue that is used to treat arrhythmias in the electrophysiology laboratory

<u>Advisory:</u> A warning issued to alert patients and care providers that a pacemaker or pacing leads may be at risk for malfunction

<u>Amplitude:</u> The level of voltage the heart generates or that a pacemaker lead delivers to the heart for pacing

<u>Anaphylaxis:</u> Severe allergic reaction

<u>Anticoagulation:</u> The amount of blood thinning present in a patient that may be on aspirin, warfarin, or heparin-based products

<u>Aorta:</u> The large vessel leaving the heart that carries blood to the rest of the body

<u>Aortic valve:</u> The valve that blood crosses when it is pumped out of the heart into the aorta

Arrhythmia: Abnormal heart rhythm that may be too slow or too fast

Asymptomatic: Lack of symptoms

Atelectasis: Minor collapse of lung airways that is common after surgeries and may cause fever or difficulty breathing

Atrioventricular (AV) node: Specialized region of tissue that conducts electrical impulses from the top heart chambers (atrium) to the bottom heart chambers (ventricles).

Atrium: The right and left atria are the top chambers of the heart and pump the blood to the ventricles

Axillary vein: The main vein that drains the arm; when the axillary vein enters the rib cage, it forms the subclavian vein

Basilic vein: This vein drains blood from the arm and joins with the cephalic vein to form the axillary vein

Bifascicular block: Electrical system block below the atrioventricular node in the right and left bundle branches

Biventricular: Refers to both the left and right ventricles and is generally used to describe a pacemaker that resynchronizes the left and right ventricles in patients with or at risk for heart failure

Bradycardia: An abnormally slow heart rate less than sixty beats per minute.

Bundle branch: The left and right bundle branches are the major branches of the conduction system that provide electrical activation for the left and right ventricles; the left bundle branch has two major subdivisions called the left anterior and left posterior fascicles

Capture: When an electrical pacing signal (voltage and current) causes atrial or ventricular tissue to contract (depolarize)

Cardioinhibitory response: A decrease in heart rate and blood pumping that can cause a loss of consciousness

Cardiomyopathy: A disease process that can cause a loss of heart muscle pumping ability and lead to heart failure

Catheter: Small tube that can be inserted in the heart via a peripheral blood vessel in the arm or leg

Catheterization: The process by which catheters are placed into the heart's chambers or coronary arteries

Cephalic vein: A large vein that is often seen in the upper arm over the bicep muscle and joins with the basilica vein to form the axillary vein; this vein runs in the groove between the shoulder and chest muscles (called the deltopectoral groove)

Chronotropic incompetence: An inability to increase heart rate during exercise or exertion

Clavicle: The medical name for the collar bone; pacemakers are generally implanted two finger breadths below the clavicle

<u>Complete heart block:</u> A complete lack of electrical communication between the atrium and ventricles that often requires a pacemaker when it is irreversible

<u>Congestive heart failure:</u> The heart cannot pump enough blood to the rest of the body

<u>Contrast:</u> Clear liquid that is used to highlight blood vessels and heart structure during pacemaker implantation

<u>Coronary artery:</u> Blood vessels that run on the outside of the heart (epicardium) and provide oxygenated blood to the heart muscle; the left main coronary artery branches into the left anterior descending and left circumflex: these generally supply blood to the left side of the heart (left atrium and ventricle); the right coronary artery generally supplies blood to the right side of the heart (right atrium and ventricle)

<u>Coronary sinus:</u> This is the major vein that drains blood from the heart muscle and directs it back toward the right atrium so blood can be reoxygenated in the lungs; the coronary sinus allows placement of pacemaker leads that are used to pace the left ventricle to enable resynchronization therapy

<u>Creatinine:</u> A blood laboratory that indicates kidney function

<u>Current:</u> Flow of electric charge through pacemaker leads

<u>Defibrillator:</u> Used to terminate life-threatening ventricular arrhythmias and requires specialized leads; all defibrillator are pacemakers, but pacemakers are not defibrillators

<u>Diaphragm:</u> This muscle is responsible for causing the lungs to expand during breathing; the phrenic nerve can be inadvertently paced causing a "hiccup" sensation

<u>Dislodgement:</u> Occurs when a lead moves out of position after a pacemaker implantation and may cause the lead to malfunction

<u>Dissection:</u> A tear in a blood vessel that may require treatment

<u>Dyssynchrony:</u> When the right and left ventricles of the heart do not contract at the same time; often present in heart-failure patients

<u>Echocardiogram:</u> A special type of ultrasound (or sonogram) that used sound waves to assess the structure and function of the heart

<u>Effusion:</u> A collection of blood or fluid around the heart or lungs

<u>Ejection fraction (EF):</u> EF is the amount of blood that is pumped by the heart during a normal heartbeat; a normal EF is between 55% and 70%

<u>Elective replacement indicator (ERI):</u> An alert on a pacemaker that signals it is necessary for the pacemaker

generator to be replaced; generally, a pacemaker can function several weeks to months once it reaches ERI

Electrocardiogram (ECG): Electrodes are placed on a patient's chest to record the electrical activity of the heart; the ECG is an important tool that cardiologists use to evaluate for disease

Electrolyte: These are elements/minerals that are found in the blood and are important for normal heart function; they can cause heart rhythm abnormalities and are measured as part of routine laboratories in preparation for pacemaker implantation

Electrophysiology: The study of heart rhythm disorders

Electrophysiology study: A procedure where a specialized cardiologist (cardiac electrophysiologist) places catheters inside the heart to record and assess the heart's electrical function

Endocardium: The inside lining of the heart muscle that is in direct contact with the blood

End of life (EOL): An alert on a pacemaker that signifies that battery is very close to empty; at EOL, the pacemaker can behave erratically and even fail

Epicardium: The outside lining of the heart that is in contact with the pericardium; coronary arteries are found here.

Erosion: Thinning of the skin over a pacemaker that can lead to infection

<u>Fascicle:</u> Branches of the heart's conduction system are called the Left Anterior and Posterior fascicles

<u>Fibrillation:</u> Very fast beating of the heart and can be seen in the atrium (not generally fatal) or ventricle (often causes death)

<u>Fistula:</u> An abnormal connection between arteries and veins that can be caused by vascular access during heart procedures

<u>Fixation:</u> Refers to how leads are attached to the heart during pacemaker implantation; active fixation involves a small helix that is screwed into the heart; passive fixation involves small, soft fingers that are wedged into the lining of the heart to stay attached (like the barbs of a fishhook)

<u>Fluoroscopy:</u> A special type of imaging that allows the doctor to perform X-rays while the patient or the heart is moving. Fluoroscopy is used during pacemaker implantation to place the leads into the heart.

<u>Header:</u> The block at the top of a pacemaker where the leads are connected

<u>Hematoma:</u> An abnormal collection of blood that can cause swelling of a pacemaker pocket

<u>Hemodynamics:</u> The study of blood flow and the body's circulation; some pacemakers have features that can detect hemodynamic indicators such as fluid retention, activity, and respiratory motion

Hemothorax: An abnormal collection of blood around the lungs in the chest that can result from a pacemaker implantation; it can be detected by a chest X-ray

High frequency jet ventilation: A special form of ventilation that is used to minimize respiratory motion during a surgical procedure

His purkinje: The fibers of the conduction system in the bottom heart chambers (ventricle)

Hydration: Refers to overall water content of a patient and the process of replacing or adding to the water content of a patient

Hypertension: Elevated blood pressure

Hyperthyroid: Abnormally elevated thyroid function

Hypotension: Low blood pressure

Hypothyroid: Abnormally decreased thyroid function

Impedance: Measure of the opposition in current that is present in the pacemaker lead

Indication: Medical reason for a pacemaker implantation

Infarction: Dead heart muscle cells caused by a heart attack; another name for a heart attack is myocardial infarction

Interrogation: The process of checking the function of an implanted pacemaker; it can be done at the bedside, in the office, or remotely while the patient is at home.

Long QT syndrome: A disease of heart muscle cells that leads to electrocardiogram abnormalities and is a cause of sudden unexpected death

Mitral valve: The one-way valve that blood crosses when traveling from the left atrium to left ventricle

Morbidity: The risk of complications, injuries, or symptoms from a pacemaker implantation

Mortality: The risk of death from a pacemaker implantation

Myopotential: An electrical potential that is created by muscle outside the heart—such as the diaphragm—that can be sensed by a pacemaker and cause a pause in pacing

Nephropathy: Damage to the kidneys

Oversensing: An abnormal detection of signals by a pacemaker that can cause malfunction

P wave: A component of the electrocardiogram that corresponds to the activation and contraction of the top heart chambers (right and left atria)

Pacemaker: A device that is used to maintain a normal heart rate

Perforation: A hole in one of the heart's chambers, arteries, or veins

Pericardiocentesis: The process of removing an abnormal collection of blood (pericardial effusion) surrounding the heart

<u>Pericardium:</u> The thin sac that lines the outside of the heart; blood collecting between the outside of the heart and this lining is called a pericardial effusion

<u>Phlebitis:</u> An inflammation or irritation of a blood vessel

<u>Phrenic nerve:</u> The nerve that controls the diaphragm

<u>Pleura:</u> Thin linings that surround the lungs and other organs inside the chest

<u>Pneumothorax:</u> An abnormal collection of air outside the lungs that can be seen after a pacemaker implantation

<u>Programmer:</u> Desktop computer that is used to interrogate a pacemaker to check function and program pacemaker features

<u>Prophylaxis:</u> A medication used to prevent a reaction or infection

<u>Pulmonary valve:</u> The one-way valve that blood crosses when traveling from the right ventricle to the lungs

<u>Pulse width:</u> The duration of the signal in milliseconds that is used to pace the heart

<u>QRS complex:</u> A component of the electrocardiogram that corresponds to the activation and contraction of the bottom heart chambers (right and left ventricles)

<u>Resynchronization:</u> Pacing feature that restores the pumping action of the heart so the right and left ventricles pump at the same time

Sinoatrial (SA) node: The natural pacemaker of the heart located in the right atrium

Sleep apnea: A sleep disorder that causes pauses or abnormally slow breathing during sleep

Stethoscope: A tool used by care providers to listen to the heart

Stroke: When blood flow to a part of the brain stops; strokes are also called transient ischemic attacks (TIA) or "brain attacks"

Subclavian vein: The vein located under the collarbone that carries blood to the heart; used to implant pacemaker leads

Supraventricular: Refers to electrical activation starting in the upper chambers of the heart (the right and left atria)

Synchrony: Simultaneous pumping of the right and left ventricles

Syncope: Loss of consciousness

T wave: A component of the electrocardiogram that corresponds to the relaxation and resetting of the bottom heart chambers (right and left ventricles)

Tachycardia: An abnormally fast heart rate above one hundred beats per minute

Tamponade: Dangerous pressure buildup outside the heart when blood collects between the outside of the heart (epicardium) and the sac that contains the heart (pericardium)

Threshold: The energy (voltage and current) required to cause the heart to beat (this is called capture)

Thrombosis: Blood clot

Tilt-Table Test: Performed to evaluate causes for syncope and involves placing a patient on a table that tilts up to a steep angle and watching for blood pressure and heart rate changes that cause symptoms

Time Out: When the doctors, nurses, technologists, and all personnel that are participating in a surgery stop what they are doing (before the patient is sedated) and identify the patient, procedure being performed (including site of implant), technique to be used, and any other important patient information (such as drug allergies)

Transient Ischemic Attack (TIA): see Stroke

Tricuspid valve: The one-way valve that blood crosses when traveling from the right atrium to the right ventricle

Twiddling: Manipulation of pacemaker or leads that may lead to malfunction

Undersensing: Failure of a pacemaker to detect native heart signals that can lead to inappropriate pacing

Vegetation: A collection of bacteria forming a mass that adheres to the pacemaker wires or inside of the heart

Vena cava: The inferior and superior vena cava are the main vessels that return the body's blood to the right atrium

Venography: An X-ray of the veins taken after contrast is injected to assess if a pacemaker lead can be inserted

Ventricle: The right and left ventricles are the main pumping chambers that pump blood to the lungs and rest of the body

Voltage: The electrical charge that can be measured or emitted by a pacemaker

Wand: A small device placed on the chest over the pacemaker and connected by a wire to the programmer; the wand enables the pacemaker to communicate with the programmer

X-ray: Special type of radiation used in medicine that is used to image bones and soft tissue

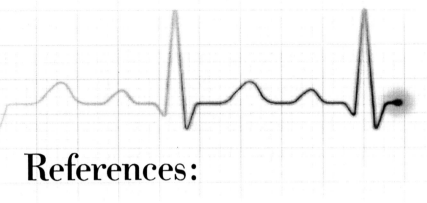

References:

1. Kurtz, S. M., J. A. Ochoa, E. Lau, Y. Shkolnikov, B. B. Pavri, D. Frisch et al. "Implantation Trends and Patient Profiles for Pacemakers and Implantable Cardioverter Defibrillators in the United States: 1993–2006." *Pacing Clin Electrophysiol*, V. 33, No. 6 (June 1, 2010), 705-11.

2. Wilkoff, B. L. "How to Treat and Identify Device Infections," *Heart Rhythm*, V. 4 (2007), 1467–1470.

3. Perls, T. "Health and Disease in People over 85," *BMJ*, V. 339 (December 22, 2009), b4715.

4. Hobbs, F. B. "Current Population Reports, Series P23-190, Sixty-Five Plus in the U.S.," accessed March 10, 2011, http://www.census.gov/population/www/pop-profile/elderpop.html.

5. Cherubini, A., J. Oristrell, X. Pla, C. Ruggiero, R. Ferretti, G. Diestre et al. . "The Persistent Exclusion of Older Patients From Ongoing Clinical Trials

Regarding Heart Failure," *Arch Intern Med*, V. 171, No. 6 (March 28, 2011), 550–556.

6. Writing Committee to Revise the ACC/AHA/NASPE 2002 Guideline Update for Implantation of Cardiac Pacemakers and Antiarrhythmia Devices, "ACC/AHA/HRS 2008 Guidelines for Device-Based Therapy of Cardiac Rhythm Abnormalities A Report of the American College of Cardiology/American Heart Association Task Force on Practice Guidelines," *JACC*, V. 51, No. 21 (May 27, 2008), e1–62.

7. Lukl, J., V. Doupal, E. Sovová, and L. Lubena. "Incidence and Significance of Chronotropic Incompetence in Patients with Indications for Primary Pacemaker Implantation or Pacemaker Replacement," *Pacing Clin Electrophysiol*, V. 22, No. 9 (September 1999), 1284–1291.

8. Lauer, M. S., G. S. Francis, P. M. Okin, F. J. Pashkow, C. F. Snader, and T. H. Marwick. "Impaired Chronotropic Response to Exercise Stress Testing as a Predictor of Mortality," *JAMA*, V. 281, No. 6 (February 10, 1999), 524-529.

9. O'Mahony, D. "Pathophysiology of Carotid Sinus Hypersensitivity in Elderly Patients," *Lancet*, V. 346 (October 7, 1995), 950–952.

10. Crilley, J. G., B. Herd, C. S. Khurana, C. A. Appleby, M. A. de Belder, A. Davies et al. "Permanent cardiac pacing in elderly patients with recurrent falls,

dizziness and syncope, and a hypersensitive cardio-inhibitory reflex," *Postgrad Med J*, V. 73 (July 1997), 415–418.

11. F. E. Shaw and R. A. Kenny. "The Overlap between Syncope and Falls in the Elderly," *Postgrad Med J*, V. 73 (1997), 635–639.

12. Curtis, J. P., J. J. Luebbert, Y. Wang, S. S. Rathore, J. Chen, P. A. Heidenreich et al. "Association of Physician Certification and Outcomes Among Patients Receiving an Implantable Cardioverter-Defibrillator," *JAMA*, V. 301, No. 16 (April 22/29, 2009), 1661–1670.

13. Cheng, A,, Y. Wang, J. P Curtis, and P. D. Varosy. "Acute Lead Dislodgements and In-Hospital Mortality in Patients Enrolled in the National Cardiovascular Data Registry Implantable Cardioverter Defibrillator Registry," *J Am Coll Cardiol*, V. 56 (2010), 1651–1656.

14. Parsonnet, V., A. D. Bernstein, and B. Lindsay. "Pacemaker-Implantation Complication Rates: An Analysis of Some Contributing Factors," *JACC*, V. 13, No. 4 (March 15, 1989), 917–921.

15. Hampton, J. R., M. J. F. Harrison, J. R. A. Mitchell, J. F. Prichard, and C. Seymour. "Relative Contributions of History-Taking, Physical Examination, and Laboratory Investigation to Diagnosis and Management of Medical Outpatients," *British Medical Journal*, V. 2 (1975), 486–89.

16. Williams, J. L. and R. T. Stevenson(2012). Complications of Pacemaker Implantation, Current Issues and Recent Advances in Pacemaker Therapy, Attila Roka (Ed.), ISBN: 978-953-51-0703-3, InTech, Available from: http://www.intechopen.com/books/current-issues-and-recent-advances-in-pacemaker-therapy/complications_of_pacemaker_implantation.

17. Tarakji, K. G., E. J. Chan, D. J. Cantillon, A. L. Doonan, T. Hu, S. Schmitt et al. "Cardiac Implantable Electronic Device Infections: Presentation, Management, and Patient Outcomes," *Heart Rhythm* V. 7, No. 8 (August 2010), 1043–1047.

18. Klug, D., M. Balde, D. Pavin, F. Hidden-Lucet, J. Clementy, N. Sadoul et al. "Risk Factors Related to Infections of Implanted Pacemakers and Cardioverter-Defibrillators," *Circulation*, V. 116 (August 2007), 1349–1355.

19. Williams, J. L., D. Lugg, R. Gray, D. Hollis, M. Stoner, and R. Stevenson. "Patient Demographics, Complications, and Hospital Utilization in 250 Consecutive Device Implants of a New Community Hospital Electrophysiology Program," *American Heart Hospital Journal*, V. 8, No. 1 (Summer, 2010), 33–39.

20. Marcos, S. K. and H. S. Thomsen. "Prevention of General Reactions to Contrast Media: A Consensus Report and Guidelines," *Eur Radiol*, V. 11, No. 9 (2001), 1720–1728.

21. Brockow, K., C. Christiansen, G. Kanny, O. Clément, A. Barbaud, A. Bircher A et al. ENDA and the EAACI Interest Group on Drug Hypersensitivity (2005). "Management of Hypersensitivity Reactions to Iodinated Contrast Media," *Allergy*, V. 60, 150–158.

22. The Royal College of Radiologists. "Standards for Intravascular Contrast Administration to Adult Patients: Second Edition," *London, The Royal College of Radiologists*, February 2010.

23. Tramer, M. R., E. vonElm, P. Loubeyre, and C. Hauser. "Pharmacologic Prevention of Serious Anaphylactic Reactions Due to Iodinated Contrast Material: Systematic Review," *BMJ*, V. 333 (September 2006), 675–678.

24. Trcka, J., C. Schmidt, C. S. Seitz, E. B. Brocker, G. E. Gross, and A. Trautman. "Anaphylaxis to Iodinated Contrast Materials:Nnonallergic Hypersensitivity or IgE-Mediated Allergy? *AJR*, V. 190, No. 3 (2008), 666–670.

25. Murkin, J. M. "Anesthesia and Hypothyroidism: A Review of Thyroxine Physiology, Pharmacology, and Anesthetic Implications," *Anesth Analg*, V. 61, No. 4 (April 1982), 371–83.

26. Farling, P. A. "Thyroid Disease," *Br J Anaesth*, V. 85, No. 1 (2000), 15–28.

27. Ellenbogen, K. A., A. S. Hellkamp, B. L. Wilkoff, J. L. Camunas, L. C. Love, T. A. Hadjis et al. "Complications

Arising After Implantation of DDD Pacemakers: The MOST Experience," *Amer J Card*, V. 92 (September 15, 2003), 740–741.

28. Link, M. S., N. A. M. Estes, J. J. Griffin, P. J. Wang, J. D. Maloney, J. B. Kirchhoffer et al. "Complications of Dual Chamber Pacemaker Implantation in the Elderly," *J Intervent Cardiac Electrophys*, V. 2 (1998), 175–179.

29. Gaitan, B. D., T. L. Trentman, S. L. Fassett, J. T. Mueller, and G. T. Altemose. "Sedation and Analgesia in the Cardiac Electrophysiology Laboratory: A National Survey of Electrophysiologists Investigating the Who, How, and Why?" *J Cardiothorac Vasc Anesth*, 2011; 25:647–659.

30. Magnusson, L. and D. R. Spahn. "New Concepts of Atelectasis during General Anesthesia," *British J Anaesthesia*, V. 91, No. 1 (2003), 61–72.

31. Lawrence, V. A., S. G. Hilsenbeck, C. D. Mulrow, R. Dhanda, J. Sapp, and C. P. Page. "Incidence and Hospital Stay for Cardiac and Pulmonary Complications after Abdominal Surgery," *J Gen Intern Med*, V. 10 (1995), 671–678.

32. Trentman, T. L., S. L. Fassett, J. T. Mueller, and G. T. Altemose. "Airway Interventions in the Cardiac Electrophysiology Laboratory: A Retrospective Review," *J Cardiothorac Vasc Anesth* 2009; 23:841–5.

33. DiBiase, L., S. Conti, P. Mohanty et al. "General Anesthesia Reduces the Prevalence of Pulmonary Vein

Reconnection during Repeat Ablation when Compared with Conscious Sedation: Results from a Randomized Study." *Heart Rhythm* 2011; 8:368–372.

34. Williams, J. L., V. Valencia, D. Lugg, R. Gray, D. Hollis, J. W. Toth et al. "High Frequency Jet Ventilation During Ablation of Supraventricular and Ventricular Arrhythmias: Efficacy, Patient Tolerance and Safety," *The Journal of Innovations in Cardiac Rhythm Management*, V. 2 (2011), 1–7.

35. Hargreaves, M. R., A. Doulalas, and O. J. M. Ormerod. "Early Complications Following Dual Chamber Pacemaker Implantation: 10-Year Experience of a Regional Pacing Centre," *Eur JCPE*, V. 5, No. 3 (1995), 133–138.

36. Noseworthy, P. A., I. Lashevsky, P. Dorian, M. Greene, S. Cvitkovic, and D. Newman. "Feasibility of Implantable Cardioverter Defibrillator Use in Elderly Patients: A Case Series of Octogenarians," *PACE*, V. 27 (March 2004), 373–378.

37. Chadha T. S. and M. A. Cohn. "Noninvasive Treatment of Pneumothorax with Oxygen Inhalation," *Respiration*, V. 44, No. 2 (1983), 147–152.

38. Kulvatunyou, N., A. Vijayasekaran, A. Hansen, J. L. Wynne, T. O'Keeffe, R. S. Friese et al. "Two-Year Experience of Using Pigtail Catheters to Treat Traumatic Pneumothorax: A Changing Trend," *J Trauma*, V. 71, No. 5 (Nov 2011), 1104-7.

39. Fyke III, F. E. "Infraclavicular Lead Failure: Tarnish on a Golden Route," *Pacing Clin Electrophysiol*, V. 16 (1993), 373–376.

40. Magney, J. E., D. M. Flynn, J. A. Parsons, D. H. Staplin, M. V. Chin-Purcell, S. Milstein, and D. W. Hunter. "Anatomical Mechanisms Explaining Damage to Pacemaker Leads, Defibrillator Leads, and Failure of Central Venous Catheters Adjacent to the Sternoclavicular Joint," *Pacing Clinical Electrophysiol*, V. 16 (1993), 445–447.

41. Belott, P. "How to Access the Axillary Vein," *Heart Rhythm*, V. 3, No. 3 (March 2006), 366–369.

42. Hirschl, D. A., V. R. Jain, H. Spindola-Franco, J. N. Gross, and L. B. Haramati LB. , "Prevalence and Characterization of Asymptomatic Pacemaker and ICD Lead Perforation on CT," *PACE*, V. 30 (January 2007), 28–32.

43. Wang, N. C,, J. L. Williams, S. K. Jain, and A. Shalaby. "Post-Pacemaker Pulsations," *Amer J Med*, V. 122, No. 4 (April 2009), 345–347.

44. Mahapatra, S., K. A. Bybee, T. J. Bunch et al. "Incidence and Predictors of Cardiac Perforation after Permanent Pacemaker Implantation," *Heart Rhythm*, V. 2 (2005), 907-911.

45. Geyfman, V., R. H. Storm, S. C. Lico, and J.W. Oren IV. "Cardiac Tamponade as Complication of Active-Fixation Atrial Lead Perforations: Proposed

Mechanism and Management Algorithm," *Pacing Clin Electrophysiol*, V. 30 (2007), 498–501.

46. Cappato, R., H. Calkins, S.-A. Chen, W. Davies, Y. Iesaka, J. Kalman et al. "Prevalence and Causes of Fatal Outcome in Catheter Ablation of Atrial Fibrillation," *JACC*, V. 53, No. 19 (May 12, 2009), 1798–803.

47. Leon, A. R., W. T. Abraham, A. B. Curtis et al.; for the MIRACLE Study Program. "Safety of Transvenous Cardiac Resynchronization System Implantation in Patients with Chronic Heart Failure: Combined Results of Over 2000 Patients from a Multicenter Study Program," *J Am Coll Cardiol*, 2005;46(12):2348–56.

48. Bristow, M. R., L. A. Saxon, J. Boehmer et al. "Cardiac-Resynchronization Therapy with or without an Implantable Defibrillator in Advanced Chronic Heart Failure for the Comparison of Medical Therapy, Pacing, and Defibrillation in Heart Failure (COMPANION) Investigators," *N Engl J Med*, 2004;350(21):2140–50.

49. D'Ivernois, C., J. Lesage, and P. Blanc. "Where are Left Ventricular Leads Really Implanted? A Study of 90 Consecutive Patients," *Pacing Clin Electrophysiol*, 2008;31(5):554–559.

50. Ellery, S. M. and V. E. Paul. "Complications of Biventricular Pacing," *European Heart Journal Supplements*, V. 6, Su D (2004), D117–D121.

51. Knight, B. P., A. Desai, J. Coman, M. Faddis, and P. Yong. "Long-Term Retention of Cardiac Resynchronization Therapy," *JACC*, V. 44, No. 1 (July 7, 2004), 72-77.

52. Jordaens, L., E. Robbens, E. Van Wassenhove, and D. L. Clement. "Incidence of Arrhythmias after Atrial or Dual-Chamber Pacemaker Implantation," *Eur Heart J*, V. 10, No. 2 (Feb 1989), 102–107.

53. Faber, T. S., R. Gradinger, S. Treusch, C. Morkel, J. Brachmann, C. Bode, and M. Zehender. "Incidence of Ventricular Tachyarrhythmias during Permanent Pacemaker Therapy in Low-Risk Patients Results from the German Multicentre EVENTS Study," *European Heart Journal*, V. 28, No. 18 (2007), 2238–2242.

54. Datta, G., A. Sarkar, and A. Haque. "An Uncommon Ventricular Tachycardia due to Inactive PPM Lead," *ISRN Cardiology*, V. 2011 (2011), Article ID 232648, 3 pages.

55. Bohm, A., A. Pinter, and I. Preda. "Ventricular Tachycardia Induced by a Pacemaker Lead," *Acta Cardiologica*, V. 57, No. 1 (2002), 23–24.

56. Freedman, A., M. T. Rothman, and J. W. Mason. "Recurrent Ventricular Tachycardia Induced by an Atrial Synchronous Ventricular-Inhibited Pacemaker," *Pacing and Clinical Electrophysiology*, V. 5, No. 4 (1982), 490–494.

57. Li, W., B. Sarubbi, and J. Somerville. "Iatrogenic Ventricular Tachycardia from Endocardial Pacemaker Late after Repair of Tetralogy of Fallot," *Pacing and Clinical Electrophysiology*, V. 23, No. 12 (2000), 2131–2134.

58. Iesaka, Y., T. Pinakatt, A. J. Gosselin, and J. W. Lister. "Bradycardia Dependent Ventricular Tachycardia Facilitated by Myopotential Inhibition of a VVI Pacemaker," *Pacing and Clinical Electrophysiology*, V. 5, No. 1 (1982), 23–29.

59. Schulza, N., K. Puschelb, and E. E. Turkc. "Fatal Complications of Pacemaker and Implantable Cardioverter Defibrillator Implantation: Medical Malpractice?" *Interactive CardioVascular and Thoracic Surgery*, V. 8 (2009), 444–448.

60. Wiegand, U. K. H., D. LeJeune, F. Boguschewski, H. Bonnemeier, F. Eberhardt, H. Schunkert, and F. Bode. "Pocket Hematoma After Pacemaker or Implantable Cardioverter Defibrillator Surgery: Influence of Patient Morbidity, Operation Strategy, and Perioperative Antiplatelet/Anticoagulation Therapy," *CHEST*, V. 126, No. 4 (October 2004), 1177–1186.

61. Sohail, M. R., S. Hussain, K. Y. Le, C. Dib, C. M. Lohse, P. A. Friedman et al.; Mayo Cardiovascular Infections Study Group, "Risk Factors Associated with Early- versus Late-Onset Implantable Cardioverter-Defibrillator Infections," *J Interv Card Electrophysiol*. V. 31, No. 2 (Aug 2011), 171–183.

62. Ahmed, I., E. Gertner, W. B. Nelson, C. M. House, R. Dahiya, C. P. Anderson et al. "Continuing Warfarin Therapy is Superior to Interrupting Warfarin with or without Bridging Anticoagulation Therapy in Patients Undergoing Pacemaker and Defibrillator Implantation," *Heart Rhythm*, V. 7, No. 6 (June 2010), 745–749.

63. Ferguson, Jr., T. B., C. L. Ferguson, K. Crites, and P. Crimmins-Reda. "The Additional Hospital Costs Generated in the Management of Complications of Pacemaker and Defibrillator Implantations," *J Thorac Cardiovasc Surg*, V. 111 (1996), 742–752.

64. Hayes, D. L. and R. E. Vlietstra. "Pacemaker Malfunction," *Annals of Internal Medicine*, V. 119, No. 8 (October 15, 1993), 828–835.

65. Alt, E., R. Volker, and H. Blomer. "Lead Fracture in Pacemaker Patients," *Thoracic Cardiovasc Surg*, V. 35 (1987), 101–104.

66. Bayliss C. E., D. S. Beanlands, and R. J. Baird. "The Pacemaker-Twiddler's Syndrome: A New Complication of Implantable Transvenous Pacemakers," *Can Med Assoc J*, V. 99 (1968), 371–373.

67. T. Fahraeus and C. J. Hoijer, "Early Pacemaker Twiddler Syndrome," *Europace*, Vol. 5 (July 2003), 279–281.

68. Ellenbogen, K. A., M. A. Wood, D. M. Gilligan, M. Zmijewski, D. Mans, and The CAPSURE Z Investiga-

tors (1999), "Steroid Eluting High Impedance Pacing Leads Decrease Short and Long-Term Current Drain: Results from a Multicenter Clinical Trial," *Pacing and Clinical Electrophysiology*, V. 22 No. 1 (January 1999), 39–48.

69. Fortescue, E. B., C. L. Berul, F. Cecchin, E. P. Walsh, J. K. Triedman, and M. E. Alexander. "Comparison of Modern Steroid-Eluting Epicardial and Thin Transvenous Pacemaker Leads in Pediatric and Congenital Heart Disease Patients," *J Interv Card Electrophysio*, V. 14, No. 1 (October 2005), 27–36.

70. Grammes, J. A., C. M. Schulze, M. Al-Bataineh, G. A. Yesenosky, C. S. Saari, M. J. Vrabel et al. "Percutaneous Pacemaker and Implantable Cardioverter-Defibrillator Lead Extraction in 100 Patients with Intracardiac Vegetations Defined by Transesophageal Echocardiogram," *J Am Coll Cardiol*, V. 55, No. 9 (March 2010), 886–894.

71. Johansen, J. B., O. D. Jørgensen, M. Møller, P. Arnsbo, P. T. Mortensen, and J. C. Nielsen. "Infection after Pacemaker Implantation: Infection Rates and Risk Factors Associated with Infection in a Population-Based Cohort Study of 46299 Consecutive Patients ," *Eur Heart J*, V. 32, No. 8 (April 2011) 991–998.

72. Nery, P. B., R. Fernandes, G. M. Nair, G. L. Sumner, C. S. Ribas, S. M. Menon et al. "Device-Related Infection among Patients with Pacemakers and

Implantable Defibrillators: Incidence, Risk Factors, and Consequences," *J Cardiovasc Electrophysiol*, V. 21, No. 7 (July 2010), 786–790.

73. Oginosawa, Y., H. Abe and Y. Nakashima. "The Incidence and Risk Factors for Venous Obstruction after Implantation of Transvenous Pacing Leads," *Pacing Clin Electrophysiol*, V. 25 (2002), 1605–1611.

74. DaCosta, S. S., N. A. Scalabrini, A. Costa, J. G. Caldas, and F. M. Martinelli. "Incidence and Risk Factors of Upper Extremity Deep Vein Lesions after Permanent Transvenous Pacemaker Implant: A 6-Month Follow-Up Prospective Study," *Pacing Clin Electrophysiol*, V. 25 (2002), 1301–1306.

75. Bracke, F., A. Meijer and B. Van Gelder. "Venous Occlusion of the Access Vein in Patients Referred for Lead Extraction: Influence of Patient and Lead Characteristics," *Pacing Clin Electrophysiol*, V. 26 (2003), 1649–1652.

76. van Rooden, C. J., S. G. Molhoek, F. R. Rosendaal, M. J. Schalij, A. E. Meinders, and M. V. Huisman. "Incidence and Risk Factors of Early Venous Thrombosis Associated with Permanent Pacemaker Leads," *J Cardiovasc Electrophysiol*, V. 15 (2004), 1258–1262.

77. Rozmus, G., J. P. Daubert, D. T. Huang, S. Rosero, B. Hall, and C. Francis. "Venous Thrombosis and Stenosis after Implantation of Pacemakers and Defibril-

lators," *J Interv Cardiac Electrophysiol*, V. 13 (2005), 9–19.

78. Worley, S. J., D. C. Gohn, R. W. Pulliam, M. A. Raif-snider, B. Ebersole, and Tuzi J. "Subclavian Venoplasty by the Implanting Physicians in 373 Patients over 11 Years," *Heart Rhythm*, V. 8, No. 4 (April 2011), 526–533.

79. Fung, J. W., J. Y. Chan, R. Omar et al. "The Pacing to Avoid Cardiac Enlargement (PACE) Trial: Clinical Background, Rationale, Design, and Implementation." *J Cardiovasc Electrophysiol*, V. 18 (2007), 735–739.

80. C. M. Yu, J. Y. S. Chan, Q. Zhang, R. Omar, G. W. K. Yip,A. Hussin,F. Fang,K. H. Lam, H. C. K. Chan, J. W. H. Fung. "Biventricular Pacing in Patients with Bradycardia and Normal Ejection Fraction," *NEJM*, V. 361, No. 22 (November 26, 2009), 2123–2134.

81. Epstein, A. E. et al. "ACC/AHA/HRS 2008 Guidelines for Device-Based Therapy of Cardiac Rhythm Abnormalities A Report of the American College of Cardiology/American Heart Association Task Force on Practice Guidelines (Writing Committee to Revise the ACC/AHA/NASPE 2002 Guideline Update for Implantation of Cardiac Pacemakers and Antiarrhythmia Devices)," *JACC*, V. 51, No. 21 (May 27, 2008), e1–62.

82. Gould, P. A. "Outcome of Advisory ICD replacement: One Year Follow-up." *Heart Rhythm* V. 5, No. 12 (December 2008), 1675-1681.

83. Carlson, M. D. and B. L. Wilkoff. "Recommendation from the HRS Task Force on Device Performance Policies and Guidelines." *Heart Rhythm*, 2006, 3:1250-1273.

84. Stevenson, R., D. Lugg, R. Gray, D. Hollis, M. Stoner, J. L. Williams. "Pacemaker Implantation in the Extreme Elderly," *Journal of Interventional Cardiac Electrophysiology*, V. 33, No. 1 (January 2012), 51-58.

Index

Author Biography

Dr. Jeffrey L. Williams is board-certified in internal medicine, cardiovascular disease, and clinical cardiac electrophysiology, and is currently medical director of electrophysiology at The Good Samaritan Hospital. He double majored in biomedical and electrical engineering at Vanderbilt University and then went on to obtain his master's degree in bioengineering from the University of Pittsburgh, where he was awarded a Keck Fellowship for graduate school. Earning his medical degree from Drexel University in Philadelphia, he then went on to complete five years of fellowship training in both cardiovascular disease and clinical cardiac electrophysiology at the University of Pittsburgh Medical Center. Possessing extensive knowledge and a unique background in both engineering and cardiology, Williams has earned numerous accolades within the academic and clinical settings, including awards from both the American College of Cardiology Foundation and the National Institutes of Health. Dr. Williams directs the only community-hospital based Heart Rhythm Center in the U.S. to publish outcomes for pacemaker and defibrillator implantations.